CANCER
Survival Guide

How to Conquer It and Live a Good Life

CANCER
Survival Guide
How to Conquer It and Live a Good Life

CHARLOTTE LIBOV

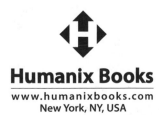

Humanix Books
www.humanixbooks.com
New York, NY, USA

HUMANIX BOOKS

DaVinci's Cancer Survival Guide
Copyright © 2016 by Humanix Books
All rights reserved

Humanix Books, P.O. Box 20989, West Palm Beach, FL 33416, USA
www.humanixbooks.com | info@humanixbooks.com

Library of Congress Control Number: 2014930398

Interior design: Ben Davis

Humanix Books is a division of Humanix Publishing, LLC. Its trademark, consisting of the words "Humanix" is registered in the Patent and Trademark Office and in other countries.

Disclaimer: The information presented in this book is meant to be used for general resource purposes only; it is not intended as specific medical advice for any individual and should not substitute medical advice from a healthcare professional. If you have (or think you may have) a medical problem, speak to your doctor or healthcare practitioner immediately about your risk and possible treatments. Do not engage in any therapy or treatment without consulting a medical professional.

ISBN: 978-1-63006-014-5 (Paperback)
ISBN: 978-1-63006-015-2 (E-book)

Printed in the United States of America

This book is dedicated to all cancer survivors
and their loved ones.

Contents

PART III — Post-Diagnosis

Foreword

MOST PEOPLE DESIRE A long life, provided they maintain their health and independence. Thanks in part to advances in medical technology, we are now living longer than ever. Most of those born in 1900 would have been fortunate to have lived beyond age 50. Today, life expectancy approaches 81 years in many countries, which has led to the greying of our population. In 2010, more than 40 million Americans were aged 65 or older — 12 times the estimate in 1900. If current trends continue unabated, we can anticipate a doubling of the number of older adults by 2030.

The goal for most of us is to achieve successful aging; we don't just want to live a long life, we want to live *well* throughout that long life. And we have made strides in achieving such quality longevity, according to the MacArthur Foundation Network on an Aging Society, which reported that genetics accounts for only about one-third of what determines wellness as people age.

Healthy lifestyle strategies and effective medical treatments can help prevent age-related illnesses, including many forms of cancer, as well as extend the number of years of successful aging.

But despite our remarkable gains in life expectancy and a greater knowledge of how to live well as we age, not everyone is living better longer. Nearly three-quarters of people aged 65 and older suffer from one or more chronic medical illnesses, such as cancer, Alzheimer's disease, Parkinson's disease, heart disease, hypertension, arthritis, and diabetes. The costs of these conditions exceeds hundreds of billions of dollars each year, and as the 78 million baby boomers begin to populate our older age group, our country must tackle a looming financial, social, and healthcare burden.

Prevention strategies can have a critical impact on many of these age-related illnesses. For example, Alzheimer's disease afflicts more than five million people in the United States, and 44 million worldwide. Although no disease-modifying treatment has yet been discovered, recent research shows that healthy lifestyle behaviors may delay symptom onset and lower disease prevalence. A new analysis estimates that nearly 50 percent of Alzheimer's cases worldwide could be attributed to modifiable risk factors, such as high blood pressure, obesity, smoking, depression, cognitive inactivity or limited education, and physical inactivity.

Many of these modifiable risk factors can prevent other diseases that burden our population at nearly every age, including heart disease, stroke, cancer, and arthritis. Remarkable medical advancements have led to effective treatment and prevention strategies for cancer, but people are not always informed about the best prevention, detection, and treatment methods available. Greater public awareness and expanded programs to help reduce smoking, increase physical activity, improve diet, and expand screening would have a considerable impact on the prevalence and mortality rate of cancer. The American Cancer Society estimates that tobacco smoking alone accounts for approximately 170,000 cancer deaths each year. In 2015, it is estimated that poor nutrition, physical inactivity, overweight, and obesity will contribute to 1.5 million cases of cancer.

When people understand the connection between their daily behavior and cancer risk, they can adjust those behaviors, lower their cancer risk, and extend their life expectancy. Legislative bodies can help to shape healthier behaviors. For instance, despite convincing evidence of the cancer risks from indoor tanning facilities, in 2013 four percent of US adults reported using such facilities during the previous year. That same year, 20 percent of female and five percent of male high school students reported using an indoor tanning device. As a result of such high usage rates, laws restricting a minor's access to indoor tanning facilities have been enacted in 42 states.

These kinds of laws will save lives, but greater awareness about the disease, its physical and psychological impact, and practical strategies for treatment and prevention are still critically needed. Those at risk for cancer or facing the challenge of a cancer diagnosis have to make difficult decisions that will impact the quality and duration of their lives. They often read conflicting accounts of "miracle cures," prevention methods, and diagnostic tests. Many people end up confused and overwhelmed by the weight of puzzling data. They need a way to put this daunting amount of complex information into perspective so they can make these vital decisions with the most rational and practical mindset, and in a very brief time frame.

The *Cancer Survival Guide* provides an informed perspective that will enlighten people at risk for cancer, patients already suffering from the disease, and their loved ones as well. By translating the latest scientific information into accessible language and practical advice, this important book will be the go-to guide for anyone navigating the threat of cancer and its consequences. Whether searching for the best doctor, deciding on an appropriate diagnostic test, or navigating the multiple options for treatment, the *Cancer Survival Guide* offers the kind of guidance that will allay anxieties and help people come up with an informed plan to deal with cancer.

Although the number of deaths from cancer has declined by 20 percent during the past two decades, scientists and doctors still have much to learn about cancer detection and treatment. While research for new treatments and cures continues, the *Cancer Survival Guide* provides an important and valuable resource for anyone desiring to live better and longer. I expect that this book's clear, sensible, and knowledgeable guidance will not only become a welcome source of information and comfort to readers, it will help extend the years of successful aging for many of them.

Gary W. Small, MD

Preface

CANCER DOESN'T WAIT.

From the instant you are diagnosed with cancer, you are bombarded with decisions that you need to make — fast. And these first steps can have huge repercussions all the way down the line, from how your cancer diagnosis is typed, sub-typed, staged, and treated, to even whether or not you survive, and your quality of life after treatment.

The problem is that you are going to be called upon to make what essentially are life-or-death decisions . . . with probably less information than you had when you decided on your last car!

The *Cancer Survival Guide* is intended to give you a jump-start in dealing with your cancer — to provide you with the tools you need to make those difficult choices, and also to quickly access additional information as you need it.

Here's just a sampling of the questions those newly diagnosed with cancer need to consider, almost instantly, or within a couple of weeks at most:

- Who is the best doctor to treat my type of cancer?

- Where can I get the best treatment?

- Should I stick with my oncologist, or visit a large-scale cancer center?

- What kind of treatment is best?

- What side effects can I expect during treatment?

- Do I need a second opinion?

- Now that I have a second opinion, whom should I trust? Do I need a third?

- What will my cancer diagnosis mean for my loved ones?

This book was written to give you tools you need to survive, and the information you need to make decisions and deal with issues that will come at you, not only in your early days as a cancer patient, but all the way through treatment and beyond.

Here's a guide to the more specific types of information you will find:

Part I: What Is Cancer?

These chapters provide you with a foundation for understanding cancer, no matter what form of the disease you have. You'll learn that there are common features that most cancers share. In addition, you'll get information on the basic tests that are used to diagnose the most common forms of cancer, and the current ways of treating cancer, from traditional surgery, radiation, and chemotherapy, to the state-of-the-art targeted treatments. In addition to conventional treatments and new therapies, you'll also find a chapter that is devoted to complementary and alternative treatments. Moreover, you'll benefit from detailed information that will guide you in choosing the best doctor and treatment center for your particular type of cancer.

Part II: Types of Cancer

This section offers vital information on the 13 types of cancers covered in this book. This includes the "big four" cancers — breast, lung, prostate, and colon — that are the most common types of cancer, comprising the vast majority of cancer cases. The remaining nine cancers may be less common, but still affect the population in great numbers; this list includes the types that are the most deadly, like brain cancer, ovarian cancer, and melanoma.

Part III: After Diagnosis

You need to educate yourself when diagnosed with cancer, and this quest doesn't end after treatment, or even years later. Part III contains information on the psychological and emotional effects of dealing with cancer through the years. In addition, you learn how cancer and its treatment will affect the rest of your body as well, so you'll be able to spot potential trouble early. Also, as a cancer survivor, you'll find tips on how to stay cancer-free for the rest of your life.

In the book's appendix, you'll find recommended reading and resources — a veritable cancer directory — meant to guide you through the process, including web addresses, physical addresses, and phone numbers for ease of use.

Throughout the *Cancer Survival Guide*, you'll meet the top doctors who are experts in your particular type of cancer, and they'll share with you their words of encouragement, guidance, and wisdom, honed from years of experience in the field. You'll also learn the inspiring stories of cancer survivors who will tell you how they did it, as well as pass their advice on to you!

On the pages that follow, you will also learn:

- The statistics and prognosis for each particular type of cancer according to the stage of the disease

- How the genes that you were born with affect your chances of getting cancer

- Exactly which types of tests are used to diagnose your specific type of cancer, and what you need to know about them

- How to choose complementary and alternative cancer treatments that work

- How to avoid the side effects of cancer treatment

- How to avoid the depression and anxiety that come with cancer

- What a cancer survivorship plan is, and why you'll need one when you finish your cancer treatment

- All about the new targeted cancer therapies that are replacing conventional treatments and when and how they can be used

- How to access clinical research studies to learn about experimental treatments that could save your life

- What future medical problems you are vulnerable to developing according to the specific type of cancer you had

- What a "patient resource navigator" is, how to get one, and how having one can help you deal with the day-to-day issues that cancer patients face

- The steps you need to take after treatment to live the rest of your life cancer-free

In short, this book has been produced to provide you with the kind of clear-cut, step-by-step tools you'll need to beat cancer. It's intended to be sharp and to-the-point. Whether you're a man or woman, or whether you are young, old, or in-between, this book is written with the fervent hope that its information will guide you in your journey from cancer patient to cancer survivor.

Acknowledgments

The author gratefully acknowledges the help of the following in the preparation of this book:

Stacey Akers, MD; Arlene Allen-Mitchell; Bruno Bastos, MD; Karen Bate; David Brownstein, MD; Nancy Butterworth; Kay Cofrancesco; Mike Craycraft; Dan Collins; Andrew Crues; Christine Darling; Annie Deck-Miller; Antonio Divine; Ginny Dixon: Joanne Filina; Juan Florez; Neil B. Friedman, MD; Robert C. Flanigan, MD; Peter Frederick, MD; David Fuehrer; Tom Halkin; Alysa Herman, MD; Elizabeth Henry, MD; Nancy Herrera; Joy Huber; Stacey Huber; Robert Kaitz; Christine Hill-Kayser, MD; Brett Johnson; Blaine Kristo, MD; Mary Leonard; John Link, MD; Nancy Link; Amy Losak; Mary Jane Massie, MD; Daryn Mayer; Jack McCallum; Ashwin Mehta, MD; Andrea Molinato; Nancy Nick; Armando Sardi, MD; Laura Porter, MD; Nancy Newsom Ridgway; Jim Ritter; Tulio Rodriguez, MD; Loretta D. Schoen; Gary K.

Schwartz, MD; Peter Shankman; Monica Smith; Patrick Stiff, MD; Anna Strazzante; Alexandra Stefanovic, MD; Dennis Tartaglia; Lee E. Tessler, MD; Jacob Teitelbaum, MD; Nora Weinstein; Jenny White; Lisa Worley; and Donald Yance Jr., CN, MH, RH (AHG).

I also want to thank all of my friends who are fighting cancer and whose stories were not included in this book, but who inspired me every step of the way, with a special heartfelt nod to Cathy Gollinger Strauss and Robert Roz Strauss.

In addition, I want to thank Travis Davis for being instrumental in matching me to this book project and to the team at Humanix Books, especially Andy Brown and Pamela Pantaleo for all their assistance throughout the shaping and editing of this manuscript.

What Is Cancer?

An Introduction to Cancer

1

JOANNE FILINA WAS 37 when she was diagnosed with a potentially deadly form of leukemia. Her doctor told her that the blood disease would probably kill her. Determined to beat the odds, Joanne decided to head to a leading cancer clinic, where she found the attitude of the doctors there to be rooted, instead, in positivity. After aggressive treatment, her cancer is now in remission.

At age 33, Mike Craycraft felt a testicular lump; his immediate thought was that he had cancer. He even made his own "bucket list," culminating in a giant good-bye party that he'd throw for himself. Although his immediate assumption was correct, today Craycraft is also cancer-free, and looking forward to many more decades ahead.

Anna Strazzante was diagnosed at the age of 41 with a potentially life-threatening and difficult-to-treat form of bladder cancer. "I felt like I'd been kicked in the stomach. It just seemed like I was living in a nightmare that I couldn't awaken from," she recalls. But today, Anna is not only cancer-free, she is a marathon runner — a sport she took up following her treatment.

Joanne, Mike, and Anna are just three of the cancer survivors you'll meet in this book. They are among the 13.7 million people living in the United States who are beating cancer. And this statistic does not include cancers that were caught in their earliest stages, so the tally is undoubtedly much higher.

If you are diagnosed with cancer today, you are more likely to survive than at any time in history. The mission of this book is to give you the tools to do it.

What Is Cancer?

Our bodies are comprised of trillions of living cells, all of which make up our organs and features — from the hair on our scalp to the toenails on our feet. These cells are preprogrammed to grow, divide into new cells, and die in an orderly fashion. Cancer takes hold when cells begin to grow uncontrollably. Instead of dying, these cells continue to grow, forming new, abnormal cells. In effect, they become immortal.

How Does Cancer Affect the Body?

In most cases, cancer damages the body because of its capacity to spread to vital organs, ultimately engulfing them and destroying their ability to perform their life-sustaining functions.

The precise way in which cancer affects the body, though, depends on the type of cancer. Most cancers are comprised of cells that clump together and form solid masses, or tumors. They spread by sending off cancerous cells that travel in the lymph system, taking up residency and colonizing in other organs. These cancers are known as "malignancies," a word that comes from Latin, meaning "to act maliciously, or with evil intent." It is an apt term.

But there are exceptions. Brain cancer, for instance, does not spread to other organs, but its growth can destroy the delicate structure within the body's vital command center. Leukemia results in armies of abnormal cells that destroy the blood's critical, oxygen-carrying function.

Major Types of Cancer

All cancers fall within one of these four major categories:

Carcinoma is the most common type of cancer. In fact, 80 to 90 percent of all cancers are carcinomas. They are solid tumors that begin in the epithelial tissue of the cells in our body, which form the covering or lining of the organs, glands, and other bodily structures. Lung, breast, prostate, colon, rectal, and pancreatic cancer, for instance, are all carcinomas.

Sarcoma begins in the connective tissue, between bones and cartilage, or in the fat, muscles, and also blood vessels. Sarcomas can develop anywhere in the body, but half of them occur in the arms and legs.

Blood cancers are those that form in the bone marrow, in the blood itself, or in the lymph system — the interconnected, cleansing superhighway that occupies spaces and vessels between tissues and organs, by which lymphatic fluid circulates throughout the body. Lymph is a colorless fluid containing white blood cells that keep the tissues healthy and free of toxins.

Central nervous system cancers begin in the tissues of the brain and spinal cord. Most of these cancers occur in or spread to the brain.

DID YOU KNOW . . .

Fifty percent of all cancers are diagnosed as one of these four major types: breast, colon, lung, and prostate cancer. All other cancers, which comprise the remaining 50 percent, are cancers that are designated as "rare" because they occur in fewer than 200,000 people a year.

Common Symptoms of Cancer

Many types of cancers have different symptoms, which occur depending on where the disease is located, its type, and how large the tumor may have grown. That said, there are some common symptoms that indicate the presence of cancer. It's important to realize, though, that many diseases, including some that are not serious, can cause these symptoms as well.

UNEXPLAINED WEIGHT LOSS

The first sign of cancer may be an unexplained loss of 10 pounds or more. This happens most often with cancers of the pancreas, stomach, esophagus (swallowing tube), or lung(s). Weight loss can also be a later sign of other types of cancers, as they rob the body of vital nutrients in order to feed their own growth. As a general rule, doctors agree that an unexplained weight loss of five percent or more of your normal body weight in a six-month to one-year period — especially for older adults — is a signal for concern and requires medical evaluation.

FEVER

A rise in normal temperature is the body's way of attempting to fight off an infection. There are several reasons why cancer can cause a fever. The body may be reacting to substances produced by the tumor, or the fever may be due to blockages the tumor causes in the kidney, bladder, or bowel. Fever can also be an early sign of a blood cancer like leukemia or a non-Hodgkin's lymphoma.

PAIN

Pain can be an early symptom of testicular cancer. A headache that does not get better with time or treatment can indicate a possible brain tumor. Back pain is not usually an early warning sign of cancer, but an indication it has spread. Such pain can be caused by colon or ovarian cancer.

SUDDEN SHORTNESS OF BREATH

Belabored breathing, wheezing, fatigue, and trouble swallowing are sometimes early signs of lung cancer.

SKIN CHANGES

Redness, swelling, dark or bruised-looking patches, or itchy skin can also be an indication of inflammatory breast cancer. Itchy skin can be a symptom of lymphoma as well. Changes in any wart, mole, or freckle, whether in color, size, shape, or border, can signal the dangerous form of skin cancer known as melanoma.

SORES THAT DO NOT HEAL

A skin cancer may bleed and resemble a sore. A long-lasting sore in the mouth could be an oral cancer. Sores on the penis or vagina are commonly caused by infection or virus, but may also be an early warning sign of cancer.

ABNORMALITIES IN THE MOUTH

White patches inside the mouth and white spots on the tongue can indicate leukoplakia, a chronic condition caused by tobacco use. If unchecked, this can become mouth cancer.

UNUSUAL BLEEDING OR DISCHARGE

Bleeding or discharge with no apparent cause should spark concern, and could signal either early or advanced cancer. For instance, spitting up blood can indicate lung cancer. Blood in the stool can be a sign of colon or rectal cancer, and uterine cancer can cause abnormal vaginal bleeding. Blood in the urine can indicate bladder or kidney cancer, and a bloody discharge from the nipple can signal breast cancer.

THICKENINGS OR LUMPS IN THE BODY

Cancerous cells clump together, so it's not surprising that many cancers can be felt through the skin. A lump is a well-known tip-off to breast cancer, of course. Lumps elsewhere in the body, especially the arms and legs, can indicate a sarcoma, which is a soft tissue cancer. Lumps in the armpit, neck, or groin area can indicate lymphoma.

INDIGESTION OR TROUBLE SWALLOWING

Persistent difficulty digesting or swallowing may be indicative of cancer of the esophagus (the swallowing tube), stomach, or pharynx (area where nasal passages connect to one's mouth and throat).

Genetics and Cancer

Cancer has always been with us. Indeed, our knowledge of cancer dates back to early recorded history. Later, the ancient Greek physician Hippocrates (460 BCE–377 BCE) gave cancer its name by describing several types of cancer with the Greek word *carcinos* (crab or crayfish) to denote the appearance of a cut, solid tumor with veins stretched out that suggested the claws of a crab to him.

The reason that cancer dates back to the birth of humankind is because it originates from deep within us — within our very genetic makeup. Deoxyribonucleic acid (DNA) contains the self-replicating genetic material, or genes, occupying every cell of our body. Our genes are arranged on chromosomes. Each cell in the human body contains 46 chromosomes, or 23 pairs, half obtained from each parent.

Here's a rundown on the types of genes involved in the development of cancer:

Proto-oncogene: These are genes that normally direct how a cell divides, but have the potential to undergo mutation and become an oncogene. The prefix "onco-" comes from the Greek *oncos*, meaning mass or tumor.

Oncogene: This is the product of a proto-oncogene that has developed a defect, mutated, and could result in a cancer. Scientists believe that we all carry oncogenes, but that they remain harmless unless triggered.

Tumor suppressor gene: These are genes we also carry that protect cells and slow their division. If something goes awry in this gene, the cancer is enabled to grow. The different genes involved in specific types of cancer are further discussed in those respective chapters.

How Genetics Works

The cells of our body contain genes that are comprised of DNA, which is known as the "genetic code," and orchestrates their functioning. The genetic code that oversees this process is contained in the 23 pairs of chromosomes; half of the code is located in a female's egg, and the other half in the male's sperm. Eggs and sperm are known as "germ cells."

When the egg and sperm meet at the moment of conception, their individual chromosomes combine to create our complete DNA code. Our DNA programs the cells to live, multiply, and then die. If, for some reason, the cell ceases to respond to the DNA's growth-inhibiting signals, it can become cancerous.

The impact of inherited genetics varies with the type of cancer. A minority of cancers — perhaps only about five to 10 percent of cancers — are directly inherited. But genetics also plays a broader role, because certain genetic mutations also increase the likelihood that a person will develop cancer. These account for cancers that seem to run in families, but do not follow the normal, direct genetic rules of inheritance.

The mutation of a gene into a cancer-causing one is not a simple process. It takes mutations in several genes for a person to develop cancer. What specifically causes mutations to occur in these genes is largely unknown. These are known as "sporadic" mutations, as they occur not due to heredity, but by chance. They may occur from aging, tobacco use, sunlight or chemical exposure, or from factors we don't yet understand, but they are not caused by genetic inheritance.

Most cancers are diagnosed in those aged 60 and older. This is because mutations in some genes become more common as we age. At the same time, aging weakens the immune process. As the immune system becomes weaker, it's less able to prevent these cancer-causing mutations from occurring.

Personal Genetic Testing

Genetic testing, which is also sometimes called "predictive testing," seeks to find specific inherited changes, or mutations, in a person's genetic makeup that could cause them to have a predisposition to develop cancer.

Even if you've been diagnosed with cancer, you should consider genetic testing for the following two reasons:

- Genetic testing can tip you off to an increased risk for developing a related form of the disease and alert you to take steps to prevent it. For instance, inheriting a BRCA gene increases the risk of developing both breast and ovarian cancer.

- Confirmation of a genetic mutation can enable you to alert your relatives that they should be tested as well, which could save their lives. There is an inherited form of colon cancer, and those people with the genetic mutation should undergo screening tests far earlier.

Currently, there are about 900 genetic tests available for all diseases, including many forms of cancer, such as breast, ovarian, prostate, endocrine, and some very rare cancers. Because of genetic trends in culture and bloodline, some individuals are highly encouraged to undergo genetic testing. For example, people of Ashkenazi (Eastern European) Jewish ancestry have been found to be at increased risk for BRCA gene mutations that cause breast and ovarian cancer. As well, testing is recommended for those with two or more family members diagnosed with the following characteristics:

- Adult cancer at an earlier than expected age (under 50)

- Developed the same type of cancer (in some cases, this might not necessarily be the exact same type, as breast and ovarian cancer can be considered the same for purposes of determining genetic predisposition)

- Two or more different cancers in the same person

- A rare cancer, such as male breast cancer or sarcoma

Lifestyle Factors That Contribute to Cancer

TOBACCO

Tobacco use is linked to 30 percent of all cancers overall and 87 percent of lung cancers. While it should come as no surprise that tobacco use is the major cause of cancer of the lungs, mouth, lips, nose, pharynx, larynx (voice box), and esophagus, it's also linked to the development of cancers of the stomach, pancreas, cervix, kidney, colon/rectum, bladder, uterus, and ovaries, as well as acute myeloid leukemia. Cigarettes are not the only culprit — these cancers are also linked to cigar and chewing tobacco use. Smokers who switch to e-cigarettes are not necessarily safe, as the risks related to this product have not yet been evaluated.

EXCESSIVE ALCOHOL USE

Not surprisingly, alcohol is a major cause of liver cancer, and the risk increases the more alcohol is consumed. But alcohol overuse is also linked to breast, mouth, pharynx, larynx, esophageal, colon and rectal cancer, and possibly pancreatic cancer as well.

OBESITY

Obesity is associated with an increased risk of cancers of the esophagus, breast (postmenopausal), uterus, colon and rectum, kidney, pancreas, thyroid, gallbladder, and possibly prostate. This is because excess body fat isn't inert. When it is located in the abdomen, for instance, it cushions the surrounding organs and produces certain hormones that may help enable cancer to thrive.

STRESS

When you talk to cancer patients, they will often trace the beginnings of their disease to a time when they were undergoing stress. But is there a true association between the two? Scientists have long tried to tease out what seems to be a connection between stress and cancer, and they've been zeroing in on two areas that may

DID YOU KNOW . . .

There are a lot of direct-to-consumer testing kits on the market, but the FDA warns these tests may not be accurate and that they could also lead people to make serious medical decisions without enough information. They also can cause people to panic. If you believe may have an inherited genetic condition, consult a qualified genetics counselor who can perform the test and also put it into perspective. See the appendix for more information.

indicate some sort of correlation there: stress on the immune system, and also the production of stress hormones, which can impact cellular growth.

It is the job of the immune system to prevent diseases like colds and flu, but it also patrols the body to prevent cancerous cells from developing. Since stress can hamper the immune system, scientists have been looking at whether this could lead to the development of cancer, but this is very difficult to prove empirically.

As well, when one undergoes stress, the body releases certain hormones including adrenaline and cortisol, which, over time, exert an unhealthy effect. Some scientists believe that the outpouring of adrenaline under stress, for instance, can cause the death of healthy cells, making way for the possible growth of cancerous ones. But this research is only in its early stages.

Stress, though, can play an indirect role, leading to cancer-causing habits like smoking, alcohol overuse, and binging on unhealthy foods packed with fat, sugar, salt, and worse; therefore, it makes sense that you should reduce your stress when it comes to not only battling the disease, but, as much as possible, preventing it in the first place.

Carcinogens and Environmental Hazards

Carcinogens are cancer-causing substances — often chemicals — that can increase a person's risk of developing cancer.

CERTAIN FOODS AND COOKING PRACTICES

Some forms of cancer can be caused by the foods we eat or the way in which they are prepared. For example, fatty foods and a lack of fiber may be linked to colon cancer, although evidence is conflicting. There is also conflicting research on grilling poultry and meats to the point of charring, so it's probably best to eat these sparingly if at all.

Additives and Preservatives

Salt and pickling are associated with high rates of cancer of the esophagus, stomach and the nasopharynx, which is the upper part of the pharynx. These cancers are rare in the United States but common in China, where salted fish and pickled vegetables are eaten in much larger quantities. Flavor enhancers like mono-sodium glutamate (MSG) and preservatives used in processed food are also suspected of causing cancer, as is recombinant bovine growth hormone (rBGH), a hormone fed to cows to increase milk production.

CHEMICALS

There are scores of chemicals known to cause cancer in humans. Some of these known and suspected carcinogens are found in the following substances:

Pesticides

Chemicals linked with the development of cancer include DDT, PCBs, and dioxin, which are found in a vast array of products, including some pesticides and lawn care products, cosmetics, and plastic bottles. Although DDT was banned years ago, the residue from it will linger forever.

Hair Dye

One-third of American women and 10 percent of men use permanent hair dye. In the past, some chemicals contained in these dyes have been linked to certain cancers in animal studies. Over the years, many of these chemicals have been removed, but there is concern about some that remain. Evidence in studies is mixed but, over the years, research has found an increase in bladder cancer in hairstylists and barbers.

CERTAIN ENERGY EMISSIONS
Sunbathing and Tanning Beds

Radiation that comes from the sun can cause skin cancer and melanoma. This is true whether the radiation comes from natural sunshine or tanning beds.

Electromagnetic Fields

It's well known that ionizing radiation, such as that emitted by X-rays and CT scans, can cause can cause cancer. But what about non-ionizing radiation, which are known as EMFs, or extremely low frequency electromagnetic fields (ELFs)? High voltage power lines, cell phone towers, home appliances, and electronics create such fields. Proponents of the theory that EMFs cause cancer point to changes in cells in test tubes and laboratory rats, but there is also evidence to the contrary as well.

Can Cancer Be Cured?

Many people who attempt to disparage our ability to cure cancer point to 1971, when president Nixon signed the National Cancer Act into law declaring a "war on cancer," and today, this disease seems as big a scourge as ever.

But this is not true. First, our understanding of cancer has increased tremendously. Although cancer was once considered a single disease, we now know that there are hundreds of different types that can all act differently, and some kinds of cancers can even seemingly transform themselves into others.

Second, we underestimated the difficulty of eradicating cancer. The biological cause of cancer is deeply rooted in our DNA, the programming that oversees the functioning of our entire body. The process that enables us to grow from babies into adults is the same process that goes awry when cancer forms.

Third, we've now seen that all attempts to find a "magic bullet" that would cure or protect us from all types of cancer have failed.

But the progress that has been made against many forms of cancer is remarkable. As you'll see from this book, cancers that were once almost sure killers, like testicular cancer, non-Hodgkin's lymphoma, and leukemia, have been transformed by time and progress into diseases that are considered either curable or manageable. The mortality rate of other types of cancers has also declined, and researchers are working diligently — and optimistically — to add more types of cancer to this list.

TIPS for Cancer Prevention

Some types of cancers are preventable. For example, not smoking, or quitting, reduces the risk of lung cancer and many other cancers as well. But the causes of a variety of cancers are not yet well-established, so information on how to prevent them is lacking. But, over the years, some clear patterns have emerged. While this book is concerned with how to survive cancer, here are the ways to help prevent the most common types of cancer from occurring:

- Don't smoke. If you do, quit. Smoking is the main cause of lung cancer and accounts for one-third of all cancers.

- Watch your weight. Excessive weight is linked to some forms of cancer, including colon and breast cancer.

- Eat a colorful diet. Fruits and vegetables that are the most colorful contain the most pigment, which makes them rich in antioxidants, protecting the body's cells from oxidation — a metabolic process that ages them and can lead to cancer. In general, rely on healthful foods for your vitamins and nutrients over supplements.

- Eat meat (especially red meat) sparingly, and avoid cured meats, like deli ham, bologna, and salami, bacon, and hot dogs. They contain nitrates and nitrites, which are linked to increased colon and stomach cancer risk.

- Enjoy a high fiber diet. While studies are mixed, the general consensus has shown that fiber may protect against colon cancer.

- Get a colonoscopy. A new study shows that colon cancer has decreased by 30 percent in the last decade, which coincided with a tripling of the rate of people getting colonoscopies.

- Exercise regularly. Physical activity not only keeps weight down and reduces stress, but also keeps hormone levels balanced.

- Consider alternative and complementary treatments along with conventional medicine but speak with your doctor first.

- Drink alcohol sparingly or not at all.

- Avoid sun exposure and tanning beds, which are both proven to cause melanoma.

- Choose organically grown fruits and vegetables.

- Avoid using pesticides in or around your home. If you must handle harmful chemicals, do so safely.

2

Diagnosing Cancer

IF TESTS INDICATE THAT you may have or do have cancer, you're probably focused on starting treatment right away. But you cannot get the right treatment — and become a cancer survivor — without having the most precise diagnosis, which will guide your doctors in treating your cancer every step of the way. This is why you need to be involved and fully invested in the diagnostic process right from the start.

It is important to remember that there is no single diagnostic test that can definitively tell whether you have cancer or not. The complete evaluation begins with a thorough medical history and physical examination, along with a series of medical evaluations.

The moment a person suspects or a doctor suggests that he may have cancer, the first inclination is usually to panic, and also quickly begin to relentlessly search the Internet. "Although there is a lot of good information on the Internet, there is a great deal of misinformation as well. People go crazy on the Internet because they see so much information that doesn't necessarily pertain to them," warns Stacey Huber, an American Cancer Society patient resource navigator at Mercy Medical Center in Baltimore, Maryland.

As difficult as it may seem, it is vital that you keep your head about you, using all of your energy to make sure that you understand every step of the diagnostic procedure all the way through.

Create a Personal Healthcare Record

A cancer diagnosis, at the very least, can be a terrifying experience. As you're being bombarded by information, opinions, and options, it is of the utmost importance that you remain grounded in order to make logical and educated healthcare decisions for yourself from the very beginning. Creating your own healthcare diary/log/record — whichever name you choose to give it — will ensure that no detail or consideration slips through the cracks to be left to chance. In a situation that would leave the best of us feeling helpless, taking authority over your healthcare will bring you down to earth, shifting your focus from that which you cannot control, to those things that you can.

"One of the most important things I learned during my cancer treatment was the importance of keeping my own medical record," says Dr. Laura Porter, a colon cancer survivor and consultant for the Colon Cancer Alliance.

There are many different tools on the Internet to help you keep a complete record of your medical care, but here's how Porter did it:

I took a big three-ring binder. On the first pages, I kept a record of my medical appointments, what the problem was, and if I had any questions for the doctor, I'd write them down there. I also had sections for all my tests and my treatment plan. In addition, I kept information about my medical history, disability, health insurance information, and legal information as well, such as documents relating to power of attorney. I also had a section where I kept the business cards of the doctors on my treatment team. I put a three-ring pencil case in the front of the binder for pens, Post-its, etc. No matter how much you'd like to think, 'Okay, I found my doctor and I'm all set,' you never know, so this is a way to keep all of your information immediately accessible.

You will see many types of doctors and all will keep separate records, so compiling your own file is the only way you will have an overview of your treatment. In addition, medical records can get lost, doctors can retire, or a new doctor you see may not receive your transferred records in a timely manner. Also, knowing the details of your treatment can help your doctor plan a new strategy should your cancer return, and this is also essential information to have if you decide you want to enter a clinical research trial.

As Dr. Porter found, keeping a complete medical record that is accurate and handy is one of the most important tools you will need, not only during your cancer treatment, but afterwards as well.

Here is a checklist from the American Society of Clinical Oncologists (ASCO) on what type of information you should include in your medical record:

✓ Your diagnosis (including specific type of cancer, stage, and areas to which it may have spread), pathology reports, and the results of any diagnostic tests performed

✓ Complete treatment information, including the names of all medications and the sites and doses of radiation therapy

✓ Treatment results, including any complications or side effects

✓ Information about any supportive care, including medication to treat pain, nausea, or other side effects that you may have experienced

✓ Information about follow-up treatments

✓ Complete contact information for your doctors and other healthcare providers and treatment centers

✓ Your family medical history

✓ Other aspects of your medical care, such as details of past physical examinations, including screening tests and immunizations

The first section of your healthcare record will be labeled "Diagnostic Testing." Use it to record any and all details regarding diagnostics, such as: the name of the test; where it was done; when it was done; who performed it; and when a follow-up test (if any) should be performed.

In addition, here are some general questions you should bring along to ask whenever a diagnostic test is recommended:

- What is the purpose of this test?

- Are there any risks or complications involved?

- Are there any alternatives to this test?

- Will I require sedation or general anesthesia?

- Is the test going to be done on an outpatient basis, or do I need to be hospitalized?

- If it is an outpatient procedure, do I need someone to drive me to or from the hospital or office?

- Is there anything that I need to do to prepare for the test beforehand?

- What is the cost involved or what cost will I be responsible for after insurance is deducted?

- When will I receive the test results?

- How can I receive a written copy of the test results?

- Will there be a follow-up consultation?

- Will there be any side effects from the test?

- Is there any follow-up testing involved?

It is important that you bring your healthcare record to each and every appointment.

General Diagnostic Tests
PHYSICAL EXAMINATION

Everyone is familiar with a physical examination. Most often it is an annual examination that is part of a general assessment of health and fitness. The doctor will take a full medical history, check your vital signs (blood pressure, heart rate, respiratory rate, and

GOOD ADVICE

As you compile your personal healthcare record, after every doctor's appointment, ask the staff for a written description of your treatment. If you're hospitalized, ask for a copy of your medical records before you leave. It's also never too late to get a record of your past treatments. Remember, you have a right to your medical records, although you may have to pay a reasonable fee (which is set by law) or wait for the copies.

temperature), listen to your heart and lungs, and examine your head and neck (this includes ears, nose, throat, eyes, mouth, and teeth) as well as check your lymph nodes, thyroid, and carotid artery. Your abdomen will also be checked, as well as your skin and the pulses in your arms and legs.

For men, a physical exam would include a check of the penis, testicles, prostate gland, and a hernia check. A woman's exam would include a clinical breast exam and could include a pelvic check as well, although this type of examination is most often performed as part of an annual gynecological checkup.

Sometimes signs of possible cancer, such as abnormal lumps or swellings, abnormal skin changes, or fever, can be detected during an annual physical examination. Most often, though, it is you who may notice symptoms and bring them to the attention of your doctor. If your doctor believes these might indicate cancer, special attention may be paid to the areas of the body involved. (See individual types of cancer.)

LABORATORY TESTS

A full blood panel, which is also part of an annual physical examination, will be performed by the doctor who will examine you for cancer. Certain lab tests that are done to check for specific cancers, such as the fecal occult stool test, which checks for colon cancer, are discussed in those chapters. However, these are two general tests that are always done as part of a physical examination:

- **Complete Blood Count (CBC):** This test checks the number of red cells, white cells, and platelets in the blood, as well as the red blood cells' oxygen-carrying capacity and the white blood cell differential, which is the percentage of each type of white blood cells present. This test can determine if an infection is present that could be causing symptoms, or if the patient is anemic, which can be a sign of cancer.

- **Urinalysis:** This involves testing the urine for different diseases, such as diabetes, kidney disease, liver disease, and urinary tract infections. This test can detect microscopic traces of blood in the urine, which could indicate bladder cancer, for instance.

ENDOSCOPY

This examination utilizes an optical telescope-like instrument called an endoscope to look inside the body. This slender tube, which is identifiable by the light on one end, can also be inserted through a small incision to obtain fluid or tissue samples to be examined under a microscope to look for the presence of cancer cells.

There are different kinds of endoscopes that can be used for different procedures: a **broncoscope** is used to check the lungs, a **cytoscope** is used for the bladder, and a **laparoscope** is used to check the ovaries, appendix, and other abdominal organs, and, as described below, a **colonoscope** is used to check the colon.

The following are some different types of endoscopies that are used to uncover problems, including cancer:

- **Upper Gastrointestinal (UGI) Endoscopy:** The tip of the endoscope is inserted in the mouth and then maneuvered down the throat, esophagus, and duodenum (upper gastrointestinal tract) to look for signs of ulcers, inflammation, infection, bleeding, or tumors. Tissue samples may also be collected. A UGI must be performed on an empty stomach, so no eating or drinking is allowed for up to eight hours before the procedure.

- **Colonoscopy:** An endoscopic procedure is done to check for polyps and cancerous tumors in the colon. The scope is inserted anally, and then slowly advanced through the rectum, into the colon. A colonoscopy requires significant preparation, including fasting and the cleansing of the colon, before it can be performed. Sedation is administered and most patients sleep through the procedure.

  There is a similar test called a flexible sigmoidoscopy, but since that procedure only allows for partial viewing of the colon, the colonoscopy has become the procedure of choice when it comes to cancer screening.

Endoscopies can also be used with other types of diagnostic tests. The **endoscopic retrograde cholangiopancreatogram (ERCP)** is a combination of two procedures: an endoscopy of the upper gastrointestinal area, which is combined with X-rays of the liver, gallbladder, and pancreas.

Endoscopy can also be combined with ultrasound for a procedure known as **endoscopic ultrasound (EUS)**. This procedure uses an endoscope that is tipped with a transducer, which converts sound waves into images. The EUS procedure can create high quality images of organs inside the body, and can also be used to check for cancerous cells in the lymph nodes — a guiding precursor to a fine needle biopsy.

CT SCAN

Computerized Tomography (CT or CAT) scanning uses computer-processed images to create photographic "slices" of the body that enable organs to be viewed in detail without having to cut into them.

In standard X-rays, a beam of energy is aimed at the part of the body being studied. A plate behind the body part captures the variations of the energy beam after it passes through skin, bone, muscle, and other tissue. While much information can be obtained from a traditional X-ray, it does not provide a detailed view of internal organs and other soft-tissue structures. In computed tomography, the X-ray beam moves in a circle around the body, which provides much greater detail. The X-ray information is sent to a computer that interprets the X-ray data and displays it on a monitor.

CT scans are used to detect lung cancer, brain cancer, and other cancers as well. It can also be used to stage cancer and help determine if it has spread or returned. By comparing CT scans over time, the doctor can also tell how the cancer is responding to treatment.

During the scan, you lie on a table that moves back and forth inside the doughnut-shaped scanner. You may have to fast in preparation. Often, orally or rectally administered (by enema), or intravenously injected radioactive contrast materials are used to produce optimal imaging. Although this material does not usually cause exceptionally adverse side effects, a tiny percentage of people may experience strong effects, such as allergic reactions.

MAGNETIC RESONANCE IMAGING

MRI is a non-invasive technique that is similar to CT scanning in that it produces high quality images of the insides of the body. Unlike CT scanning, though, it does not use radiation. Instead, this technology uses superconductive magnets and radio waves to obtain its image.

For this test, you lie motionless on a scanner table, which again, like the CT, is drawn slowly into a huge, similarly doughnut-shaped machine. Although this test does not involve any pain, it can be uncomfortable to those who are prone to claustrophobia. Magnetic resonance imaging can be used in the diagnosis of several types of cancer, including breast cancer.

GOOD ADVICE

Since the MRI is basically a magnet, some people worry that if they have a pacemaker, a mechanical heart valve, or artificial hip, it may not be safe for them to undergo this procedure. This varies, depending on the implanted device, so you should inquire about it beforehand.

CHEST X-RAY

Painless and noninvasive, chest X-rays create pictures of the structures protected by your ribcage, such as your heart, lungs, and blood vessels. This is one of the oldest of diagnostic tests, dating back to 1895, but is still very widely used today to detect a large variety of diseases, including cancer. The test is easily administered, and no preparation or sedation is needed; you simply stand against the film cassette and pictures of your chest are taken from different vantage points. The procedure takes only about 15 minutes.

POSITRON EMISSION TOMOGRAPHY

This test, commonly known as **PET** scanning, is another accurate way of envisioning the inside of the body without the use of invasive procedures. The PET scanner, like many of the other imaging devices, looks like a huge doughnut; you lie on your back on a table that is inserted into the doughnut's hole. A small amount of radioactive isotope is injected into your body. As the isotope decays, or loses energy, it emits small particles called positrons, which can be detected as they leave the body. The scanner detects this substance to produce sharp, three-dimensional images of the inside of the body. Because cancer cells tend to use more energy than healthy cells, they absorb more of the radioactive substance, and thus appear exaggerated in the scan's results.

INTEGRATED PET-CT SCAN

In this case, the scans are done at the same time using the same machine, then the results are combined. The CT scan provides detailed pictures of the tissues and organs, while the PET scan shows any abnormal activity that may be occurring within them. Currently this combination technique is being used in the diagnosis, staging, and monitoring of melanoma, breast, esophageal, lymphoma, lung, colorectal, head and neck, and ovarian cancers.

CYTOLOGY

Cancer is almost always diagnosed cytologically — by studying cells under a microscope to determine if any are cancerous. The cells that are used for this examination are generally those that have been shed or shaved off of living tissue, or are contained in fluids, like sputum, which is used to check for lung cancer. Cytology can also be used to test cells obtained from the breasts, spinal cord, prostate or thyroid, as well as the bone marrow. Among the most familiar of cytology tests is the Papanicolaou test (named for the Greek doctor who invented it), widely known as the Pap smear, which is used to check for cervical cancer, among other diseases and infections.

DID YOU KNOW . . .

The American Society of Clinical Oncology recommends that follow-up PET or PET-CT scans not be given to patients who have finished treatment that was intended to eliminate the cancer. According to the organization, such repeated testing has not been found to save lives and may subject patients to unnecessary treatment, as well as needless cost and worry.

BIOPSY

Generally, a physical examination, blood tests, and many of the other diagnostic tests discussed in this chapter can suggest that cancer is present, but often the only true confirmation of a cancer diagnosis can be obtained solely through a biopsy.

When performing a biopsy, a small amount of tissue is removed and the results examined under a microscope by the pathologist (physician who interprets changes and diagnoses disease found in tissue and body fluids) in order to determine whether the sample contains benign (noncancerous) or malignant (cancerous) cells. In cancers such as leukemia, the cells are evaluated via a microscopically examined blood smear. The results of a biopsy can also be used to stage the disease.

There are many different types of biopsies, depending on the nature of the potential cancer. They include:

- **Fine needle aspiration biopsy:** The doctor uses a very thin needle to pierce the skin and collect a small amount of fluid and cells. This is best for smaller tumors, especially if they can be felt through the skin.

- **Core needle biopsy:** This procedure is similar to a fine needle biopsy, but uses a larger needle to extract a larger portion of tissue. The advantage is that the larger tissue sample will provide the pathologist with more information about the possible tumor.

- **Vacuum-assisted biopsy:** This type of biopsy uses vacuum pressure (suction) to collect a tissue sample through a specially designed needle. This procedure allows for the collection of samples from larger or multiple biopsy sites.

- **Image-guided biopsy:** This method combines the use of imaging technology (like the CT scan, ultrasound test, or MRI) with the biopsy procedure. The imaging tests are used to pinpoint the exact location of the tissue that needs to be removed for biopsy, and then any of the other biopsy procedures described in this section can be performed to remove it.

- **Surgical biopsy:** The surgeon makes a cut in the skin and removes some or all of the suspicious tissue. It is usually performed after a needle biopsy shows cancer cells, but can be used from the beginning to obtain a diagnosis. It may even be a treatment if all the cancerous cells can be removed.

BONE SCAN

This diagnostic is used to detect bone cancer or to learn if another type of cancer has spread (metastasized) to the bones. A form of nuclear medicine, bone scans utilize a small amount of injected radioactive material, which attaches to the bones in order to allow for imaging.

Generally, no special preparations are needed. At the start of the test, as the radioactive "tracer" circulates through your body, you will need to drink water so any of the excess tracer material that does not accumulate in your bones can be excreted. You then lie on your back on an exam table while a large scanning camera mounted above moves slowly across your body, taking a full skeletal survey. You can resume your normal activities following the test.

Cutting-Edge Diagnostics

Tumor marker testing is a newer form of screening that is playing an increasing role in the modern diagnosis, treatment, and management of cancer.

The concept of tumor marker analysis is fairly simple: The doctor takes a sample of tumor tissue or bodily fluid (such as blood, urine, or stool) that could contain tumor markers, and sends it to a laboratory where it is analyzed. This analysis involves checking for substances that are produced by cancer cells, or other bodily cells' response to cancer. Normal cells also manufacture tumor markers; however, cancerous cells produce them in far higher quantities.

Most tumor markers are proteins, though more recently, genetics has begun playing a role, as patterns of gene expressions and changes in DNA can be found in some types of tumor tissue.

Tumor markers can be measured before treatment begins to determine which treatments will be most successful, or they can help determine the stage of the disease or the patient's prognosis. They can also be used to monitor the patient's response to treatment, and to determine if the cancer has returned.

Given that conditions other than cancer can affect a person's tumor markers, they are generally not enough to base a diagnosis upon, but are used in conjunction with other tests, like imaging procedures and biopsies. Thus far, about 20 clinical markers for tumors have been characterized and are in regular use.

GOOD ADVICE

The use of tumor markers and genetic testing is the wave of the future and will someday enable the targeted treatment of more types of cancer without the toxic side effects of chemotherapy. Therefore, you should have your tumor's markers checked and the information recorded, because even if there is no clinical treatment for your type of cancer now, there may very well be if your tumor should return in the future, for instance. Be sure to discuss options with your doctor, as new tumor markers are always being discovered.

Diagnostic Testing and Radiation

Radiation is a known cause of cancer and many of the tests discussed in this chapter, including the chest X-ray, CT scans, and nuclear medicine tests (such as PET scans and bone scans) emit radiation. (MRI and ultrasound exams do not use ionizing radiation.)

The need for accurate diagnosis is generally thought to outweigh the risk; however, it is not surprising that concern has mounted among those who are healthy as well as cancer sufferers, who are exposed to far higher radiation levels than ever before.

Over the years, radiation-based diagnostics have proliferated. In 1990, fewer than three million nuclear studies were performed in the United States, but this number more than tripled by 2002. In 2007, it was estimated that 72 million CT scans were performed in the United States annually, and researchers at the National Cancer Institute estimate that this degree of testing may actually cause 29,000 future cancer cases — a figure that does not include the potential risk from other types of radiation-emitting tests. The Susan G. Komen foundation has also found radiation from such testing to be an environmental cause of breast cancer.

To protect yourself as much as possible, here are some questions to ask to make sure that you will receive the lowest amount of radiation possible when undergoing tests:

QUESTIONS TO ASK

- Is this test necessary? What will you learn about my medical condition that you could not find out by other means?

- Are you ordering this test in accordance with the recommendations established by the leading clinical guidelines?

- Are there any alternatives that don't utilize radiation that can provide you with the information you need?

- Is the facility that is administering the test able to adjust the protocol to suit the individual needs of each patient? (I.e., if an identical protocol is used for each patient, there may be a missed opportunity to lower the level of radiation that is used.)

- Will the equipment that is to be used emit the lowest amount of radiation possible? For instance, a newer CT scanner, known as the "Ultrafast," can deliver a lower amount of radiation than those that are called "spiral" or "multi-detector" CT scanners. Sometimes the type of test requires a CT scanner that emits a higher level of radiation; however, this is not always the case.

- If the test uses injected nuclear materials, will they be of the type that emits the lowest amount of radiation or can the lowest amount be used that will not affect the quality of the test results?

Along with the previous list of questions, this list should also be kept in the "Diagnostic Testing" section of your personal healthcare record.

Cancer Treatments

3

THE ROOTS OF MODERN cancer treatment reach back to 1846, when anesthetic practices became widely utilized in the Western world, and surgery to treat cancer became feasible. The first mastectomy was performed in 1882. Radiation therapy can be traced back to the discovery of X-rays in 1895, and the development of chemotherapy dates back to World War II.

It may not seem that much has changed — conventional cancer treatment still relies on the same basic methods: surgery, radiation, and chemotherapy. But a revolution in cancer treatment is underway, utilizing targeted treatments that are more effective and cause fewer side effects.

First we will focus on those long-established treatments, followed by the targeted treatments. Bear in mind that the course of cancer treatment you receive will depend on factors specific to your case. These may include the following:

- The type/nature of your cancer

- The stage of the cancer

- Whether the cancer is newly diagnosed or has recurred

- Any additional medical conditions that you have, whether cancer-related or not

Questions to Ask Your Doctor

Before getting started, you'll want to create the next section of your healthcare record, labeled, "Treatment." Record the following questions to ask your doctor about treatments that may be considered for your particular type of cancer:

- What are my treatment choices?

- What factors did you take into consideration when making this recommendation?

- Why is this treatment preferable to other treatments?

- What's the goal of the treatment?

- How will we know that the treatment is working?

- What are the benefits and risks of this treatment?

- Could this treatment cause other health problems over time?

- How will my daily life be affected?

- Will I still be able to work while I am under treatment?

- Are there any treatments that might be preferable at a major cancer center?

- Whom would you recommend for a second opinion?

Types of Treatment
SURGERY

In many cases, the first line of cancer treatment is the removal of the mass or affected area. Surgery is most effective on small tumors, or tumors that are localized to a specific part of the body. Sometimes, especially in the case of cancers that are discovered early, surgery is all that is needed to cure the disease.

Often, surgical procedures are combined with other treatments, such as chemotherapy, radiation, or hormonal treatments to reduce the risk of recurrence (commonly used for breast and prostate cancers). Historically, surgery is the oldest treatment for cancer and it is still the one most commonly used, both to cure cancer and sometimes if the disease recurs. Surgery is generally not used if the cancer is advanced and has spread to other organs.

Surgery is generally performed in a hospital or surgical center under anesthesia, and preparations, length of hospital stay, and recuperation vary depending on the type of surgery involved. All surgery carries some risk, including infection, blood clots, and also the potential removal of an organ, which can produce side effects. The outcome also depends on several factors, including the health and condition of the patient, the skill of the surgical team, and the facilities.

A very important term you'll hear in connection with cancer surgery is **clear margins**. When the surgeon removes the tumor, tissue samples from the same site are also taken and examined for cancer cells. If the surrounding area is free of cancer, this is the best indication that the disease has not spread.

Sometimes, surgery will still be warranted even though clear margins cannot be achieved. In such cases, a surgical procedure called **debulking** may be used instead. This refers to removing as much of a malignant tumor as possible, so that chemotherapy and/or radiation will be more effective. Debulking, or **cytoreduction surgery**, is often used in the case of brain or ovarian cancer.

CHEMICAL TREATMENT

Chemotherapy is the use of specific chemical agents or drugs that target cancer cells. It can be used before surgery, but most often it is used afterward or in conjunction with radiation. While it can cure some types of cancers that have spread within the body, it is also used to eradicate any cancerous cells that may remain after surgery. In addition, it can be used to control the growth of cancer if it returns. For some

GOOD ADVICE

If you've been told you are a candidate for surgery, check out the doctor's credentials. The best choice is usually a surgeon who is board-certified, a Fellow of the American College of Surgery, and who is experienced in performing the type of surgical procedure you need. Also, a top surgeon usually has a top-flight surgical team, which is important as well.

cancers, chemotherapy is given as a "maintenance" therapy to help keep the disease in check.

Rapidly dividing cells are a hallmark of cancer. However, not all cells that grow quickly are necessarily cancer. Chemotherapy cannot differentiate — it also kills healthy cells, like the ones that cause hair growth, or those that line the mouth and intestines. This causes the unpleasant side effects for which chemotherapy is known: hair loss, nausea, and vomiting. Most of these side effects improve or disappear after the chemotherapy is stopped; but some types of chemotherapy can permanently damage the heart, lungs, and other organs.

The type of chemotherapy used depends on the kind of cancer you have, how advanced the disease is, and your general physical condition (whether you have any other medical conditions, such as heart or kidney disease, etc.).

There are different ways to administer chemical therapy, but it is most often given intravenously. It is also usually given in cycles with rest periods in-between, which enable the body to recover and grow new, healthy cells to replace those that were eradicated during the cancer treatment.

Heated Chemotherapy

Hyperthermic intraperitoneal chemotherapy (HIPEC), known as a chemo bath, is an aggressive form of chemotherapy and surgery given to patients with advanced cancer who may have run out of treatment options. This two-step procedure, which is performed in one lengthy operation that can last several hours, can be used on cancers that have spread to the abdominal wall, such as late-stage colon cancer, and those of the appendix and stomach.

First, the surgeon removes all visible signs of tumor with cytoreductive surgery. Then, the chemotherapy drug, cisplatin, is heated to 103 degrees Fahrenheit and pumped into the abdominal cavity. The patient, who is lying on a cooling table, is physically rocked back and forth to make sure the chemical mixture is spread throughout the abdomen, killing any remaining cancer cells. The entire procedure can last from eight to 18 hours.

Significantly riskier than conventional treatments, the extreme nature of this procedure has stirred considerable controversy due to a lack of studies proving its effectiveness. However, a study published in 2013 in the journal *Cancer Medicine* looked at 112 patients with very advanced colon cancer. One-half of the patients were treated with this method, and the remaining half with conventional chemotherapy. According to the results, this procedure was no more risky than the conventional treatment, and one in three patients survived at least five years, compared to a survival rate that is usually measured in months.

Heated chemotherapy is a highly involved and extremely invasive treatment with potentially severe toxic effects, so it should only be performed by an exceedingly skilled surgical team on carefully selected patients.

RADIATION

Cancer treatment using high-energy X-rays or similar high-energy (ionizing) particles — radiation therapy — has been in practice for over 100 years. There are two main forms of radiation: external radiation involves receiving treatment from outside the body, with the use of a machine; internal radiation, known as **brachytherapy**, is performed by placing radioactive material inside the body, into the cancer itself or the tissue surrounding it.

Like chemotherapy, radiation has the same drawback — this treatment also can kill healthy cells nearby, as well as causing side effects. Therefore, other forms of radiation systems are being developed in order to kill cancer cells while sparing as much healthy tissue as possible. They include:

- **Intraoperative radiation therapy:** Radiation is delivered directly to the tumor during surgery. The surgeon finds the cancerous cells, moves normal tissue out of the way, and then focuses the radiation on them.

- **Systemic radiation therapy:** Radiation is delivered orally or intravenously using agents known as radioactive pharmaceuticals. The drugs then travel through the body, targeting cancer cells.

- **Radioimmunotherapy:** A radioactive agent is combined with a monoclonal antibody, which is then injected or infused into the body. Monoclonal antibodies mimic those produced by our bodies; they attach to the cancer cells, marking them so that the defective cells are identified for removal by the immune system. Since the antibodies guide the solution directly to the cancer cells, healthy tissues are spared.

- **Proton therapy:** Also known as "proton beam" therapy, this type of radiation uses positively charged particles (protons) instead of x-rays to treat cancer. Protons can destroy cancer cells while emitting less radiation, which means that more healthy tissue is spared. This may translate into lesser side effects as well. Additionally, proton therapy is more focused treatment than general radiation, making it particularly valuable in treating cancers that are deep within the body and have not spread. Proton therapy has been found particularly useful in treating sarcoma, and its use is being pioneered in breast, lung, prostate, and other cancers.

Targeted Therapies for Cancer

Although surgery, chemotherapy, and radiation are still the dominant forms of cancer treatment, more and more targeted therapies are being developed to treat different forms of cancer. This is the long-awaited revolution in cancer treatment, and it is no longer the "future" of cancer therapy — it's our present reality!

These targeted therapies do not treat cancer as broadly as surgery, chemotherapy, or radiation, but they are specialized treatments that block the spread of cancer by interfering with specific molecules involved in tumor growth and progression.

These drugs, too, have a drawback, though — they don't work for all types of cancer or even on all cancers within a certain type. They only work on tumors or cancer cells that have

GOOD ADVICE

While targeted therapies do not yet exist for all forms of cancer, this is the hottest research field. So if you need more effective treatment and no targeted therapies exist for your type of cancer, there may be work underway. This is a good reason to seek out a clinical trial.

characteristics such as certain hormone receptors or genetic markers.

There are different types of targeted therapies, so this section contains a general rundown of them.

HORMONE TREATMENT

Hormones are chemicals produced by glands in the body. There are many types of hormones, but two major are involved in cancer treatment: estrogen, which is produced primarily by the ovaries, but also found in small amounts in men; and testosterone, which is mainly manufactured by the testicles, as well as being found in lesser amounts in women. These hormones oversee development and functioning of the body's reproductive organs, but they can also fuel the growth of some types of cancer.

Hormone therapy means manipulating the amount of these hormones in the body, either by adding or reducing certain ones in order to kill cancer cells or halt their proliferation. This type of therapy can be used alone or in conjunction with other treatments.

Not all cancer tumors respond to hormone therapy, so to find out if yours does, your doctor will recommend a hormone receptor test. This test measures the amount of certain proteins (hormone receptors) in the cancer tissue. If the test results are positive, then hormone therapy can be used to treat the cancer cells.

Hormone therapy can be administered in many ways. Most of the time it involves taking medications that stop or block the production of the hormones. Surgery can also be performed to remove the gland that is producing the hormones. In addition, hormone therapy has proven useful in preventing cancer; for instance, tamoxifen can be used both to treat breast cancer and to prevent it in women at high risk for the disease.

IMMUNOTHERAPY

Also know as "biological treatment" or "biologics," immunotherapy is a type of cancer treatment that marshals your immune system to fight cancer. Some of these agents use living organisms, substances derived from them, or synthetic versions of such substances to accomplish this.

Although the immune system is known primarily for fighting off infections one of its most important functions is to protect the body by killing cells that become cancerous. This is not a foolproof system, however. Your body is programmed to recognize any substance that is foreign, or believed foreign (like germs), and set off an alarm, creating antigens to attack it. But cancer cells can fool the immune system. In addition, it grows weaker as we age, a reason most cancer occurs in those 60 and above. Immunotherapy is designed to bolster the immune system's cancer fighting power.

The following are different types of biological treatments:

GOOD ADVICE

If you have a type of cancer for which immunological treatment is not stipulated, check further. As of this writing, there were several agents in the process of clinical trials, so it's wise to check every so often.

- **Monoclonal antibodies (mAbs):** When the immune system detects antigens it produces antibodies to combat them. These mAbs bind to the antigens that are on cancer cells, but not on normal and destroy cancer cells by eliciting an immune response.

- **Cytokines:** These are signaling proteins that white blood cells produce. They aid in communication between cells to trigger the immune system should a pathogen be detected. Cytokines also combat inflammation and promote the formation of new blood cells.

You may recall hearing about the cytokine **interferon (IFN)**, which was the anticipated wonder drug for cancer treatment. Those hopes didn't pan out, but interferon has proven to be valuable in the treatment of some forms of cancer. Another cytokine, interleukin, can be used in this manner. A third type, hematopoietic growth factors, help lessen the side effects of some types of chemotherapy and boost bone marrow function.

- **Gene therapy:** This treatment attacks cancer at its root the gene mutations that set off uncontrolled cell growth that defines cancer. This therapy delivers altered genetic material to the patient to replace the defective genes that caused the cancer. Such therapies are still being developed, but they are among the most promising treatments underway. It is hoped that gene therapy will someday supplant drugs and surgery.

- **Cancer vaccines:** Cancer-specific vaccines are another highly anticipated cure, utilizing potential agents that stimulate the production of antibodies to provide immunity against a number of cancers. Progress in this arena is beginning to materialize, and there is now a vaccine that fights metastatic prostate cancer (prostate cancer that has spread). FDA-approved vaccines that indirectly fight cancer include one that guards against human papillomavirus (HPV), accounting for 70 percent of cervical cancer cases, and another that fights the hepatitis B virus, which is known to cause liver cancer. Vaccines for most major forms of cancer are currently undergoing clinical trials.

BONE MARROW/STEM CELL TRANSPLANTATION

A bone marrow transplant (known also as a stem cell transplant) is a very aggressive way of treating cancers, particularly those types that don't form solid tumors. These include leukemia, multiple myeloma, and some types of lymphomas, including non-Hodgkin's.

Bone marrow is the soft, flexible tissue that fills the cavities of our larger bones; the stem cells in bone marrow are responsible for the manufacture of red blood cells, platelets, and most white blood cells. The goal of the bone marrow or blood stem cell transplantation in leukemia, for instance, is to replace the diseased or nonfunctional stem cells with healthy stem cells. A bone marrow transplant can also enable a person to undergo chemotherapy at higher doses than that which would ordinarily damage the bone marrow.

"This type of procedure was once used to treat advanced breast cancer, but it did not prove to be effective; however, there are currently some programs that are looking at treating testicular and ovarian cancer this way, but this is not standard treatment," says Dr. Tulio Rodriguez, medical director of bone transplantation at Loyola University Medical Center.

"When it comes to bone marrow transplantation, patient selection is very important," notes Dr. Rodriguez. "These treatments are usually reserved for younger patients, as opposed to those who are elderly, but there is also a 'gray area,' so patients should be carefully screened." In addition, the center should have a good cancer survivorship program so patients can be followed for complications for the rest of their lives. "Some people withstand a bone marrow transplant with minimal discomfort, while others may have complications throughout their life, so patients need to be prepared for this," he adds.

CLINICAL TRIALS

Before a new drug or other type of cancer treatment goes on the market, the Food and Drug Administration (FDA) must grant it approval. In order to gain approval, the treatment must pass through a multi-phase research study during which it has been tested on human subjects to prove safety and effectiveness. This is where you, the cancer patient, come in.

When it comes to clinical studies, many are under the impression that this is a treatment option of last resort. In reality, though, clinical trials are a valid and viable option, especially when we consider that cancer drugs available today made their way to the marketplace via this same rigorous testing process. For example, there may be courses of treatment being studied that have fewer side effects or are easier to tolerate than those on the market. When battling cancer, it is crucial not to discount any possible treatment alternatives. An excellent resource is CureLauncher.com, an Internet-based, personalized service that matches patients with research studies.

Pharmaceutical and other types of medical companies are constantly seeking patients for clinical trials. But finding the right trial can be daunting. Traditionally, the way to find a trial was to go through ClinicalTrials.gov, a site run by the National Institutes of Health, which lists all clinical trials underway; however, a current look found more than 163,000 trials underway throughout the United States, as well as in 185 other countries.

At any given time, there are 10,000 trials in the United States enrolling patients: 4,000 for cancer, 500 for breast cancer, 50 for testicular cancer, and so on. With such numerous opportunities, it's no wonder that patients aren't being referred to clinical trials, because doctors simply don't have the time to learn about them.

Especially in the case of advanced cancer, patients may be understandably reluctant to enroll in a double-blind study. In such a study, half of the patients receive the therapy, and the other half receives a placebo, or an inactive treatment; for those desperately seeking life-sustaining, medical intervention, being placed in a placebo group compromises their very precious time. In the case of CureLauncher, if a patient has no interest in a placebo study, the service will find them one that ensures the individual will get the treatment. Alternatively, a cancer patient may be worn out from the toxic effects of chemotherapy and is seeking a gentler treatment. CureLauncher will also factor this in when matching a patient with a clinical study.

Internet search sites for clinical trials are popping up, but Cure-Launcher differs from these because, from the moment a patient clicks on the website, a window opens and a person is greeted by a relationship manager who offers them help. These relationship managers are not simply computer-generated, customer service reps, but real people who are trained to sort through all the possible clinical trial opportunities and match the patient with the best possible option.

Because of its approach, the health outcome is so much better — instead of being a company that markets a trial, CureLauncher starts out with one person and matches them to any one of the clinical trials, and this creates a better experience for the patient.

Clinical trials are divided into specific, defined phases. Contrary to what many people believe, most clinical trials have already completed their earlier stages, such as animal research projects, and are in the latter stages of testing, when large-scale enrollment begins.

Here's a rundown of the phases of a clinical trial:

- **Phase I:** An experimental drug or treatment is tested in a small group of people (20 to 80) for the first time to evaluate safety and side effects.

- **Phase II:** The drug or treatment is administered to a larger group of people (100 to 300) for further evaluation.

- **Phase III:** The drug or treatment is administered to large groups of people (1,000 to 3,000) to confirm effectiveness, monitor side effects, compare it with standard or equivalent treatments, and collect further information.

- **Phase IV:** The FDA has approved the drug or treatment and it is now on the market. But research will continue to track its safety, seeking more information about a drug or treatment's risks, benefits, and optimal usage.

The following are questions, provided by the Center for Information & Study on Clinical Research Participation, which you

should include in your healthcare record and ask when you are considering participating in a particular clinical study.

QUESTIONS TO ASK

• What is the main purpose of this study?

• Does the study involve a placebo (inactive treatment) or a treatment that is already on the market?

• How will the treatment be administered?

• How long is the study going to last and what will I be asked to do as a participant?

• What has been learned about the study treatment and are any study results published?

• Do I have to pay for any part of the study? Will my insurance cover these costs?

• Is there any reimbursement for travel costs or childcare?

• Will I be able to see my own doctor?

• If the treatment works for me, can I keep using it after the study?

DID YOU KNOW . . .

Many people are skeptical of clinical trials because they fear that they are conducted without respect and consideration for individual needs — that they will be treated as mere guinea pigs. This is not the case. The FDA monitors all phases of a clinical trial. Participants are protected by the same legal and medical code as in all areas of medicine. People also can opt out of a clinical trial any time they wish.

• Can anyone find out whether I'm participating in the clinical trial?

• Will I receive any follow-up care after the study has ended?

• What will happen to my medical care if I stop participating in the study?

• Does the physician/investigator have any financial or special interest in the clinical study?

• What are the credentials and research experience of the physician and study staff?

To find other helpful Internet sites for clinical trials, refer to the appendix.

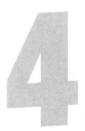

Alternative Cancer Treatments

WHEN BRETT JOHNSON WAS diagnosed with an oligodendroglioma — a particularly fierce type of brain tumor — he decided to marshal every weapon he could against it. To treat the tumor, he turned to surgery, radiation, and chemotherapy at Dana-Farber Cancer Institute, one of the nation's top cancer centers. He also cast a wide net for ways to nourish his mind and soul as well.

Johnson employed healing modalities like meditation, acupuncture, and color visualization. But he was also aided in many ways by the other techniques, including asking those who would be treating him to say certain mantras. "As crazy as it sounds, it helped," he says.

When faced with cancer, many patients turn to treatments outside mainstream medicine. Whether you call it alternative, natural, or holistic medicine, Americans spend $34 billion a year on it, and one survey shows that about 65 percent of Americans diagnosed with cancer have used such methods, compared to 53 percent of the general population.

Traditionally, such treatments have gotten a bad rap from the scientific community, especially when they are considered in place of Western medicine. But one of the biggest trends in cancer treatment today is the blending of traditional medicine with non-mainstream modalities under the umbrella term of "integrative medicine."

Before getting into that, though, here's a rundown on the terminology:

- **Alternative medicine:** This generally means the use of non-mainstream approaches in place of conventional medicine.

- **Complementary medicine:** The term describes the use of non-mainstream therapy in conjunction with traditional, Western-style medicine. Alternative and Complementary Medicine are often referred to together under the acronym "CAM."

- **Integrative medicine:** This approach to healing combines treatments from standard medical care with complementary approaches, for which there is high-quality evidence of safety and effectiveness.

A great deal of confusion exists in the use of these terms, so don't be surprised to hear complementary and integrative medicine being used interchangeably , along with CAM!

One of the forces leading the way in this field is the National Institutes of Health, which is an agency of the US Department of Health and Human Services. The NIH established the National Center for Complementary and Alternative Medicine (NCCAM) with the goal of subjecting such approaches to rigorous scientific studies.

Another excellent resource is the Society for Integrative Oncology (SIO), which aims to advance evidence-based, comprehensive, integrative healthcare in order to improve the lives of people affected by cancer.

Both NCCAM and SIO offer workbooks for patients who want to talk to their doctors about integrative care. (See the appendix for resources.)

Who Pays for These Treatments?

Whether or not health insurance will pay for nontraditional therapies depends on your coverage. If the treatments are hospital-based, the cost may be covered as part of your hospital care. Many therapies may not be covered by traditional healthcare insurance, but are considered a medical expense so they may also be eligible under a healthcare flexible spending account.

Alternative Philosophies in Practice

DR. ASHWIN MEHTA

Director of Integrative Medicine at Sylvester Comprehensive Cancer Center at the University of Miami's Miller School of Medicine, Ashwin Mehta, MD, believes in treating the whole person using an arsenal of tools that integrates Eastern philosophies into Western medicine.

"When you talk about alternative versus conventional medicine, there is an unfortunate connotation that you have to choose one or the other. I don't believe that cancer patients should have to make such a choice," says Dr. Mehta.

At the Sylvester Comprehensive Cancer Center, patients are educated about holistic measures that can complement treatment. This includes recommendations from physicians, dieticians, exercise physiologists, and there is also an acupuncturist on the staff.

"If cancer is a weed and the body is the garden, then it's the job of the surgeon, the oncologist, and the radiologist to eradicate the weed. But once treatment is completed, it's our job to strengthen and nourish the garden to minimize the chance of the cancer coming back," says Dr. Mehta.

"Often, patients ask their oncologists questions about nutrition, exercise, mindfulness techniques, and other types of additional therapies they wish to pursue, but their doctors don't have answers for them. In this case, integrative medicine can fill that gap."

When it comes to nutrition, for instance, cancer patients are recommended to follow a low glycemic diet — a diet low in sugar and carbohydrates that avoids insulin spikes. According to Mehta, "Cancer cells replicate faster than normal cells. They have the ability to grab onto sugar particles in the bloodstream and are more adept at soaking up easy sugars, so one of the things we do is encourage clients to be mindful about how much sugar they are taking in."

"Patients are also urged to stay away from processed, under-cooked, and raw meats, and lean toward fruits and vegetables and other foods that strengthen the immune system," says Dr. Mehta. "The nutritionist also guides patients toward foods that inhibit the body's inflammatory response, which can be aggravated due to chemotherapy," he adds.

"We also teach cancer patients how to do mindfulness meditation, because studies say that people who are regular practitioners strengthen their immune system, and the immune system can unleash natural cells that kill cancer," Mehta believes. "These are just some examples of how integrative practices can help fight cancer," he notes. In addition, all patients at the center are screened for depression, sleep problems, and given an exercise prescription as well as recommendations on vitamins and supplements.

"I'm very open-minded," says Dr. Mehta, who trained at Dr. Andrew Weil's Center for Integrative Medicine at the University of Arizona. "For us to recommend a therapy, it has to be evidence-based; it has to have been validated in clinical trials. If a patient has advanced disease, we may be a little more cavalier, but for someone who has a good prognosis and is receiving treatment, we want therapies that are solid and evidence-based because we want to go for a cure," he says.

Dr. Mehta's department, like most other integrative cancer centers, offers services along these lines:

- Herbal medicine consultation
- Nutritional counseling
- Physical activity/exercise counseling
- Meditation, yoga, and tai chi classes
- Education in restful sleep practices
- Acupuncture
- Art therapy
- Animal-assisted therapy
- Music therapy

GOOD ADVICE

Acupuncture, the Chinese practice of inserting needles into the skin at particular points, is a popular alternative treatment. If you or a loved one are considering acupuncture as an alternative therapy, it is important to realize that those undergoing cancer treatment are especially likely to have weakened immune systems, so it is vital that acupuncturists use sterile needles. The practitioner should use new disposable (single-use) needles for each patient, the National Institutes of Health notes.

DONALD YANCE, CN, MH, AHG

"Herbal treatment is the oldest medicine in the world," says Donald R. Yance, Jr., co-author of *Herbal Medicine, Healing & Cancer: A Comprehensive Program for Prevention and Treatment.* Yance, a certified nutritionist and master herbalist, has created a system that he calls the "Eclectic Triphasic Medical System (ETMS)," which is both a diagnostic and therapeutic system for the care of the whole person. He also runs the Mederi Foundation and the Mederi Centre for Natural Healing in Ashland, Oregon.

Yance's approach is a blend of science along with many other modalities, including traditional Chinese and Ayurvedic (traditional Hindu) medicine. His system incorporates the following fields:

- Botanical medicine
- Nutritional medicine
- Dietary medicine
- Lifestyle medicine
- Pharmaceutical medicine

Yance includes the term "triphasic" in his system, as this program of care encompasses the three main dynamics of self — the body, the mind, and the spirit — but also takes into consideration the individual, the environment, and the disease process. He thoroughly assesses each patient (or host) as well as the cancer.

"We evaluate the person based on an energetic assessment by looking at the life force, which includes the five organ networks, the inner system of the person, and their symptoms. In addition, we look at the person's microenvironment, which is influenced by the host and the cancer, with our goal of making it the most hospitable to the host and the least hospitable to the cancer," he says.

"When you are diagnosed with cancer now, you are still going to get the same standard treatment, usually chemotherapy. That is the standard of care. We do a lot of testing, including blood tests and genetic tests, to arrive at the person's particular genotype (their genetic inheritance), and then we hit that genotype with particular botanical compounds that target those particular genetic markers," he says.

This customization of therapy is important so that when traditional cancer treatment such as chemotherapy is needed, it can be employed at the lowest possible dosages for the least toxicity. He also believes that a variety of healing methods, such as healing work, should be used to strengthen the person as much as possible so that eventually the cancer is weakened, loosens its foothold, and is eventually banished.

DID YOU KNOW . . .

Memorial Sloan Kettering Cancer Center has created a free app called "About Herbs" to provide cancer patients with information on herbal botanicals, supplements, and complementary therapy. The app is available for iPhone, iPad, and iTouch devices. Download it from the Apple App store. There is a non-Apple web application as well. (See the appendix for more information.)

DR. JACOB TEITELBAUM

Affectionately known as "Dr. T.," Jacob Teitelbaum, MD, is a board-certified internist and medical director of the Practitioners Alliance Network. He is the author of several books, including *Real Cause, Real Cure*, which discusses natural cures for cancer. He believes in a "comprehensive" approach to treating cancer, which incorporates both natural medicine as well as science-based therapies.

"I realize it is hard to know what to do when your oncologist (and most that I've met are incredibly caring and well-meaning) criticizes natural therapies on one side, while your natural doctor believes that chemotherapy is killing you. The premise of 'Comprehensive Medicine' is to use the best of natural and prescription therapies, and applies brilliantly to treating cancer," says Dr. Teitelbaum.

One of the issues with alternative cures is the lack of scientific data supporting them, but this is not surprising, considering the costs (and profit) involved in bringing new pharmaceutical drugs to market.

"The FDA approves drugs not by how effective or worthwhile [they are], but whether they can show a statistically significant difference between placebo and the actual medication. The medication may add a week to your life, but make you sick as a dog and cost you $150,000. The doctors say we have to do something and they make their money giving the medication, so this results in a strong bias toward chemo," he notes.

Dr. T. strongly believes that antioxidant supplements can help lessen the effects of chemotherapy, and he cites a 2008 study that looked at the effects of glutathione, melatonin, vitamin A, N-acetylcysteine, vitamin E, selenium, L-carnitine, coenzyme Q10, and ellagic acid on patients taking chemotherapy. "Five of the studies found that subjects taking antioxidants were able to complete more full doses of chemotherapy," he says.

He notes that some oncologists believe that antioxidants can decrease the effectiveness of chemotherapy and radiation, so in these cases, Dr. T. discontinues them for a week before or after treatments if the oncologist is concerned.

"I have found that trying to starve you [in order] to starve and kill the cancer cells is a losing proposition in the long term. People do best when their own defenses are kept strong, so they can remain vital and otherwise as healthy as possible while the prescription medical treatments are doing their job," he says.

In addition, he also recommends to all his cancer patients a special highly absorbable type of curcumin, which he says research shows has been getting good results and is now being studied for a variety of different types of cancer.

Dr. Teitelbaum suggests patients ask these questions of their oncologists:

- How big a difference will this medication make in my treatment?

- How likely is it that I will respond to it?

- How toxic is it?

- What are the likely side effects?

- Do you know of any natural alternatives that have been shown to be helpful?

- Would combining natural or alternative treatments interfere with the standard therapy and, if so, is the conflict in concurrent treatments documented?

Dr. Teitelbaum also offers a free app entitled "Cures A–Z" that is available for both iPhone and Android models. Check your phone's app store.

DR. DAVID BROWNSTEIN

David Brownstein, MD, is a board-certified family physician, one of the foremost practitioners of holistic medicine, and the medical director of the Center for Holistic Medicine in West Bloomfield,

Michigan. He also writes the *Natural Way to Health* newsletter for Newsmax Media.

Dr. Brownstein believes that nutritional deficiencies, especially those involving iodine, are a chief cause of cancers that arise from the body's glands, which are the most common types, including breast, colon, lung, and prostate cancer.

"Your body is like an intricate, finely-tuned machine with tens of thousands of working parts. Some of the most important parts are essential nutrients, enzymes, and hormones. But everything is connected, and one part depends on another for normal and healthy body function," says Dr. Brownstein.

"When you're young, everything works fine, but with aging and toxin exposure due to the environment, this hormonal balance is thrown out of whack, leaving you more susceptible to disease — including cancer."

Iodine is one of the most important nutrients because every cell in the body uses it, especially the white blood cells, which are part of the immune system and the body's first defense against cancer. He also contends that the government sets the RDA, or recommended daily allowance, of iodine too low.

"We've got a very serious iodine deficiency in our country, which is one reason I believe we're seeing increases in breast and prostate cancers, as well as no reduction in the death rates," states Brownstein.

According to Dr. Brownstein, he (and his partners) have tested more than 6,000 patients and found 96 percent of them to be iodine deficient. In one study, he also found that breast cancer patients had iodine levels 50 percent lower than his average female patients without breast cancer.

"People who are iodine deficient get cysts on their glandular structures, and those cysts become nodular. If this continues, they take on the appearance of hyperplasia, which is pre-cancer, and the next stage is cancer. The interesting thing about iodine is that it's been shown in animals and test tubes to not only stop, but also reverse this continuum. I've seen this happen in my patients as well," he says.

Dr. Brownstein recommends the following steps to cancer patients — and non-cancer patients — to counteract an iodine deficiency:

- Get your iodine level checked and if it is too low, take an iodine supplement of 12 to 50 milligrams.

- Clean up your diet and rid it of anything with toxic chemicals, particularly products that contain brominated flour or vegetable oil. Bromide (found in many home products), blocks the absorption of iodine.

- Use unrefined sea salt instead of conventional table salt.

For a more extensive discussion of Alternative Medicine for Cancer, and additional physician listings, see Appendix B.

TIPS Regarding Alternative Cancer Treatments:

Should you decide to pursue any non-mainstream cancer treatments, here are some important points to keep in mind:

- Do not use any of these therapies as a substitute for conventional cancer care. There is no scientific evidence that such therapies alone cure or prevent cancer.

- Ask about the benefits, risks, and side effects of the particular therapy.

- Make sure you inform your doctor of any of these therapies that you are considering. Some herbs and dietary supplements may affect how conventional treatments like chemotherapy and radiation work, and could lessen their effectiveness or cause an adverse reaction.

- Don't abandon your natural sense of skepticism. If something seems too good to be true, it probably is.

GOOD ADVICE

While there is no shortage of well-meaning healthcare practitioners, there are also individuals out there who prey on those they believe vulnerable, and cancer patients fall into this category. Two watchdog organizations to check with before making your decision are the National Council Against Health Fraud, or NCAHF.org, and QuackWatch.com.

How to Choose a Doctor and Hospital

5

WHEN DIAGNOSED WITH CANCER, you will be instantly faced with what may seem like countless decisions to make. Choosing a doctor and hospital will undoubtedly be the most important of these decisions — and of your life, for that matter — yet many people just go along with the first recommendation they are given by the diagnosing physician. Doctors often bristle that people put more work into choosing a car than they do into selecting a physician; sadly, they are right.

Sometimes, immediate treatment is necessary, but in most cases, you do have the time to do a little research and make an informed decision on which doctor should oversee your care and where you should be treated.

Some people choose their doctor first, while others choose the cancer treatment center. There is no right or wrong way to approach this. Often, the doctor who ends up heading your cancer treatment team will be one referred to you by your internist or primary care doctor. If you are comfortable with that doctor and his or her qualifications, this may work out very well. But if you are not, or if you are referred to more than one specialist, you may very well need to go about your own selection process.

Selecting Your Doctor

There are three major types of oncologists, and based on their titles, their functions are rather obvious, but it's worth mentioning in order to get you to begin considering all of the pieces of the cancer-care puzzle.

MEDICAL ONCOLOGISTS

The most general type of cancer doctor, these physicians specialize in diagnosing and treating the disease by using chemotherapy, hormonal therapy, biological therapy, and targeted therapy. During your treatment, you may very well see different types of cancer specialists, but your medical oncologist will often be your main medical provider and should be considered the "captain" of your medical team.

SURGICAL ONCOLOGIST

Biopsies and, of course, surgical procedures are the main responsibility of the surgical oncologist. The biopsy is one of the most important diagnostic tests you'll undergo, as it can lead to the correct staging and treatment for your particular cancer.

RADIATION ONCOLOGIST

If radiation should be part of your cancer treatment plan, this medical professional would perform it. Radiation is a very important procedure that carries risks similar to surgery, and so you select your radiation oncologist with the same care as your surgeon. This statement seems obvious — that one would select any of one's healthcare practitioners with an equal degree of care — but with so many decisions to make, it's sometimes easier to go on recommendation rather than putting forth the effort to research.

"Generally, your best choice is a doctor who has the most experience treating the specific type of cancer you have. Usually, such doctors are found in the nation's top cancer centers, although this isn't always so," says Dr. Lee Tessler, neurosurgeon and executive director of the Long Island Brain Tumor Center. "Clearly, you need the best team, but you don't want your doctor 500 miles away. You want to be able to call your oncologist or surgeon and get an appointment to come in without a long wait," Dr. Tessler adds.

The oncologist to whom you are referred may turn out to be the right doctor for your case, or you might decide to seek another. Again, this is one of the most important choices you'll need to make, and it is solely in your hands. Below are organizations with searchable online databases that can help you find a doctor or do a credential check. For further information on how to contact them, refer to the appendix.

- American Society of Clinical Oncology (ASCO), ASCO.org
- American Board of Medical Specialties (ABMS), ABMS.org
- American College of Surgeons, FACS.org
- American Medical Association, AMA-ASSN.org

How to Choose a Treatment Center

These days, cancer treatment centers abound, and these facilities, whether large or small, are all using slick marketing strategies. When you are diagnosed with cancer, your inclination may be to drop everything and head for one of these branded centers. This may or may not be the right choice for you.

"On one hand, the top cancer centers are now more accessible than ever, and many people don't realize that you don't need connections to go to them. On the other hand, a smaller hospital nearby may be better for you as long as the expertise is there because during cancer treatment, having friends and family on hand to support you can give you the all-important boost you need," notes colon cancer survivor, Dr. Laura Porter.

"During the first year of my colon cancer treatment, I was never alone. I had people coming from Baltimore a couple of times a week, I had friends who would take off work — my cousin's wife, my sister — they all came to sit with me so that I wasn't alone," Porter recalls.

CANCER CENTERS OF EXCELLENCE

The National Cancer Institute (NCI) has a program that identifies the best cancer facilities in the United States. There are three designations within this program:

- Comprehensive Cancer Centers
- Cancer Centers
- Basic Laboratory Cancer Centers

GOOD ADVICE

If you have a rare form of cancer — one that is particularly difficult to treat — or you are at high risk due to age or complicating medical conditions, you may do best at an NCI-designated treatment center due to their multidisciplinary approach.

NCI-DESIGNATED COMPREHENSIVE CANCER CENTERS

This top designation given by the NCI recognizes facilities for both the superiority of their treatment and the breadth of the programs they offer. They are also acknowledged for their research programs in innovative cancer care. As of this writing, 41 of the 68 NCI-designated cancer care centers were comprehensive treatment centers.

NCI-DESIGNATED CANCER CENTER

As with comprehensive cancer care centers, these facilities are recognized for the expertise of their doctors in addition to their work in the forefront of cancer research.

And again, like comprehensive cancer care centers, these facilities must also excel in the following areas:

- Multidisciplinary, state-of-the-art treatment
- Expertise in rare cancers
- Clinical trials and other research studies
- Outreach, education, and cancer control programs

These centers are also very prestigious, so they draw top cancer experts from around the world and they also see large numbers of patients with all different types of cancer.

NCI-DESIGNATED BASIC LABORATORY CANCER CENTERS

These centers do not provide patient care, but only conduct cancer research. There are currently seven NCI-designated basic laboratory centers.

ACCREDITED CANCER TREATMENT HOSPITALS

There are 1,400 hospitals and medical centers accredited by the Commission on Cancer (CoC) of the American College of Surgeons. This voluntary accreditation program is designed to ensure that patients at these centers receive the following services:

- Quality care close to home

- Comprehensive care offering a range of state-of-the-art services and equipment

- A team approach to coordinating the best cancer treatment options available

- Access to cancer-related information and education

- Access to patient-centered services that include psychological screening

- Genetic assessment and counseling services

- Pain management services

- Treatment based on national treatment guidelines

- Information about clinical trials

- A plan for follow-up care designed for cancer survivors

- Lifelong patient follow-up

GOOD ADVICE

These days, terminology similar to "cancer center of excellence" and "comprehensive cancer center" are used by many hospitals for marketing purposes, but they don't necessarily denote NCI-designated programs, so make sure to do your research.

NATIONALLY ACCREDITED PROGRAM FOR BREAST CENTERS (NAPBC)

The NAPBC is a program to identify and recognize breast cancer treatment centers in the United States. A consortium of leading health organizations chooses those facilities that meet the program's 28 standards and 17 components. These treatment centers are deemed to provide the most efficient and contemporary care available for patients diagnosed with diseases of the breast. The components include meeting certain criteria in terms of diagnostic testing, staging, medical oncology, nursing, education, outreach, quality improvement, cancer survivorship programs, radiation, and plastic surgery, among other facets of care. For treatment centers that meet NAPBC requirements, check the appendix.

Second Opinions

There are many reasons for wanting to get a second opinion. You may be newly diagnosed and seeking confirmation that your doctor's recommendations are the best. Or you may have concerns about your current treatment and want to explore other options.

"There is nothing more that I want to tell people than not to be afraid to make a change," says Joanne Filina, mother of two who was diagnosed with chronic lymphocytic leukemia at age 37.

"I know how hard it is to leave a doctor. I stayed with my family doctor for two years before he finally did tests that gave me a diagnosis, and then he referred me to a specialist who told me I had 18 months to live. My husband said, 'I will fly you to China if I have to.' I didn't have to do that, but I did go to see another specialist and that was a whole different ball game," says Filina.

Many people worry that their doctor will be offended about getting a second opinion, but if this is the case, that might be a tip-off that a second opinion is needed. If the second doctor's opinion is different from the first doctor's and you are still uncertain, you can go back to your family doctor for advice, or you can seek a third opinion to see if there is a consensus from two of the doctors as to which treatment course is best.

The Role of the Patient Navigator

If you are a newly diagnosed cancer patient, you may feel that your whole world has changed. That's understandable, because in essence, it has. But what can really help you through the process is having a skilled professional by your side. This is where the American Cancer Society's (ACS) Patient Navigator program comes in.

"Usually at that first appointment, patients are overwhelmed. They have seen three or four doctors, and they have so much on their plate they just can't even take anything in. We are here to help guide them, so they don't have to go through this alone," says Stacey Huber, an ACS cancer navigator at Mercy Medical Center in Baltimore, Maryland.

This is a free service sponsored by the ACS, and is offered in most cancer centers. There are individuals who perform similar functions, but go by other names, such patient advocates or hospital social workers. Whatever they are called, these are people who can help you through your treatment, assisting you in finding the help you need, whether it is financial support, insurance, transportation, caregiver support, or even just to lend an ear — right from the start.

"If you've been newly diagnosed, ask the hospital what they have to offer. Ask for any and all support services that they offer. Set up a meeting with them and listen to what they have to say," says Huber.

Financial issues are often among the top concerns of patients. "A lot of people are in the middle-class income bracket; they have mortgages, utilities, two kids, and they may be out of work while they are being treated, so they are only getting 60 percent of their paycheck and the costs can add up," she notes. This adds to the stress, so Huber helps her clients work out payment plans and find whatever financial help is available.

In addition, such an advocate can help you in talking with your spouse, children, and relatives about cancer and refer you to support groups for these topics.

So when you are facing a cancer diagnosis, reach out. Find a patient navigator, advocate, or caseworker. You don't have to handle it all alone.

QUESTIONS TO ASK

The following are questions to consider when choosing a doctor:

- What are the doctor's credentials?

- Does the doctor have experience treating my form of cancer? How many cases of this type of cancer does the doctor treat each year?

- Is the doctor affiliated with the hospital or treatment center of my choice?

- How long does it take to get an appointment?

- Is the doctor or another healthcare professional accessible to me if I have questions between visits?

- Who covers for the doctor when he or she is unavailable?

- Does the doctor have access to clinical trials?

- Does the doctor take my private health insurance or accept Medicare patients?

- Does the doctor seem encouraging, interested, and respectful?

PART II

Types of Cancer

6

Breast Cancer

SURVEYS SHOW THAT WOMEN consider breast cancer their biggest threat. This is not surprising, since breast cancer is among the most common of cancers — every woman personally knows someone who has had it. The disease carries the threat of not only death, but also disfigurement.

Time for a reality check! Breast cancer is indeed common, but if you get this form of cancer, you are more likely to survive it, as Nora Weinstein learned. Although she lost her grandmother and aunt to the disease and her mother battled it as well, today Weinstein is a breast cancer survivor. "There have been so many advances in the field of breast cancer that I feel very positive going forward," says Weinstein, who was first diagnosed two decades ago and is now 70 years old.

What Is Breast Cancer?
Like other cancers, breast cancer begins when normal cells change and grow uncontrollably, forming a tumor. A tumor can be benign

(noncancerous) or malignant (cancerous, with the possibility of spreading to other parts of the body). Some breast cancers are localized, meaning they are confined to the breast. When malignant, the cancer tends to spread to the bones, lungs, and liver, or, less often, to the brain.

Statistics

With the exclusion of skin cancer, breast cancer is the most common form of cancer in US women. An estimated 300,000 women will be diagnosed with breast cancer this year; this includes roughly 235,000 cases of invasive breast cancer (the type capable of spreading), and 65,000 of breast cancer *in situ* (from the Latin for "localized"), or the type that is not yet capable of spreading. About 40,000 American women die from the disease each year.

To better understand these statistics, the numbers show that about one in eight women will develop breast cancer, which is just under 12 percent of the population. This translates to about 125 new cases for every 10,000 women in the population.

After lung cancer, breast cancer is the second most common cause of cancer-related death in women. However, since 1990, the number of women who have died of breast cancer in the United States has steadily decreased, and today, 90 percent of those diagnosed are expected to survive for at least five years.

Most women who develop breast cancer are 60 years of age or older — a fact often overlooked because breast cancer victims as portrayed in the media tend to be much younger. However, young women are more likely to die from it.

About 20 percent of women with newly diagnosed breast cancer have a family history of the disease. This means having a first-degree relative (mother or sister), a second-degree relative (niece, grandparent, or half-sister), or a third-degree relative (first cousin or great-grandmother) who had breast cancer. Some genetic syndromes also raise the risk of ovarian cancer, so knowing your family history in that regard is important as well.

When you are assessing your genetic risk of breast cancer, don't just focus on your maternal history (mother's side of the family).

You received half of your genes from your father, so the women on that side of the family count as well.

Outcome and Survival Rates

There are nearly three million breast cancer survivors in the United States.

Localized breast cancer, which is a small tumor(s) confined to one area of the breast, has a 98.6 percent cure rate. If the cancer has spread to another area within the breast, that survival rate drops to about 84.4 percent. But, as mentioned previously, even the nearly one-quarter of women with late-stage breast cancer survive five years or more.

"Today women are living longer as survivors of breast cancer. I have had the privilege to care for women with breast cancer for 30 years and have seen the overall cure rate increase from 55 percent to close to 90 percent," says Dr. John Link, one of the world's leading breast cancer oncologists and author of *The Breast Cancer Survival Manual*.

DID YOU KNOW . . .

Women who develop breast cancer in one breast are at an increased risk of one to two percent per year for developing cancer in the opposite breast, even if they have no other breast cancer risk factors.

In addition, treatments today are less drastic than ever. Dr. Link continues: "I tell women that our top priority is to cure you, and that our secondary goal is to allow you to survive with the best quality of life and to return you to normalcy, and this is what happens in the vast majority of cases."

Types of Breast Cancer

There are many different ways of classifying breast cancer. The most common way used to be classifying it according to where the cancer occurred, and then determining how likely it was to spread. According to this classification system, most breast cancers fell into one of two types: **ductal carcinoma**, which occurs in the cells lining the breast ducts, and **lobular carcinoma**, which occurs in one or more of the breast's 15 to 20 lobes.

You'll still often find breast cancer classified this way, but genetic analysis has transformed the way it is staged and treated. This is why each breast tumor is subject to genetic testing. "It helps that a woman's breast cancer be classified as one of four types, instead, which helps her and her doctors plan a more precise strategy," says Dr. Link.

"Determining the type of cancer you have is critically important because your treatment course depends on it," emphasizes Dr. Link. For instance, luminal A cancers can often be cured primarily with limited surgery and radiation, but chemotherapy is generally not needed. On the other hand, chemotherapy is a main treatment for luminal B cancers. "But even the aggressive cancers are yielding to new treatments," he notes. "The HER2-type used to be the worst type of cancer, but now we have Herceptin and other drugs, which have raised the cure rate from 57 percent to the low 90s. We are thinking that eventually, it's going to be curable," Dr. Link adds.

LUMINAL A

This is a type of slow-growing, low-grade cancer, and the type most commonly discovered by mammogram screening. The outcomes are excellent, and the cure rate is more than 90 percent. These cancers all have estrogen and progesterone hormone receptors on the cell surface, which means they are easy to treat. They do have to be treated, though, because of the possibility that luminal A cells can change into luminal B cells.

LUMINAL B

These cells are more aggressive than luminal A. They are estrogen receptor positive, but often lose the progesterone receptor from the cancer cell surface. They also have the potential to spread to the lymph vessels.

TRIPLE NEGATIVE

Known also as "**basal type**" breast cancer, it is referred to as "**triple negative**" because the tumors don't have estrogen or progesterone receptors, or evidence of the HER2-positive gene. These tumors account for 20 percent of all breast cancers, and they also tend to be fast growing, spreading, and aggressive. They are more common in younger women, and in those women who are carriers of the BRCA1 gene.

HER2-POSITIVE

About 20 percent of breast cancers overproduce a gene called the HER2 oncogene, which is a powerful, cancer-causing gene that sends messages to the cells to grow and spread.

Rare Breast Cancers Types

The four types of breast cancer cited above comprise the vast majority of breast cancer cases, but there are rare breast cancers as well. Of these many rare forms of breast cancer, two of the most common types are **inflammatory breast cancer** and **Paget disease** of the breast (or nipple).

INFLAMMATORY BREAST CANCER

IBC is an aggressive form of breast cancer, with symptoms that include a thickening and reddening of the skin over the breast. This aggressive, fast-spreading cancer, which was once almost always fatal, is now showing much better cure rates when treated aggressively with chemotherapy prior to surgery, Dr. Link says.

PAGET DISEASE OF THE BREAST OR NIPPLE

Named for 19th-century British doctor Sir James Paget, this is a rare cancer in the skin of the nipple or in the skin closely surrounding it. This form of the disease is usually, but not always, found with an underlying breast cancer. About one to three percent of breast cancers are Paget disease of the breast.

Genetics and Breast Cancer

Nancy Herrera was just turning 50 when she went for her routine mammogram. She was getting ready to go on a trip in a few days when she received the letter. "They said it was an abnormal reading, so they wanted me to come back," she recalls. But, since Nancy had been religious about going for screenings, and there was no history of breast cancer in her family, she didn't worry about it at all. But, on the second visit, the doctor told her they needed to do a biopsy. She underwent the procedure. "They told me I had ductal carcinoma in situ (DCIS). After that, everything went very fast."

DCIS is really considered a pre-stage cancer finding, and sometimes it does not require treatment at all, only monitoring. But every case needs to be considered on an individual basis, and in Nancy's case the diagnosis resulted in the removal of both of her breasts, and her ovaries as well. This is because Nancy was born with the BRCA1 gene mutation — a mutation that dramatically raised her risk of both breast and ovarian cancer.

The discovery of the **BRCA1** and **BRCA2** gene mutations in the 1990s transformed our knowledge of breast cancer. Women who carry the BRCA1 mutation, which is the primary one, account for only two percent of the population, yet they have a 70 percent increased lifetime risk of developing breast cancer. Not only that, but if they do develop breast cancer, it is far more likely to be triple negative — an aggressive and very difficult type to treat.

Nancy's discovery that she was a BRCA1 carrier completely changed the picture of her breast cancer diagnosis. In fact, she'd been found to be a carrier years earlier when undergoing genetic testing during pregnancy, but the finding wasn't pertinent at the time, so she had completely forgotten about it.

DID YOU KNOW . . .

The BRCA genetic mutations are not the only ones linked to increased breast cancer risk. There are additional more newly discovered genetic mutations, including one known as PALB2. The PALB2 gene is called a "partner" gene to BRCA because it works with it, but this is a far more rare mutation.

"The discussion went from 'we can do a lumpectomy' to 'we are going to have to do a mastectomy and a full hysterectomy as well.' I was shocked. I remember that first day when I was telling my family and I was crying so hard I couldn't talk," recalls Herrera.

Since then, she's undergone the mastectomy and the hysterectomy as well as breast reconstruction, and she is looking forward to a healthy life "I'm healed. I still have to go for regular checkups, but I'm fine," she says.

A decision to undergo a prophylactic, or preventive, mastectomy and hysterectomy is controversial, but not unusual, especially for BRCA1 carriers.

Unlike those diagnosed with breast cancer, there is a classification called **previvors**, which is the name given to women who are born with a strong hereditary risk of breast and ovarian cancer but haven't yet developed the disease. Depending on their individual case, their options range from screening to tamoxifen therapy, or even prophylactic mastectomy. One famous previvor is Angelina Jolie, whose preventive mastectomy made headlines.

But with proper treatment, even women who have BRCA1 cancer do not necessarily face a shorter lifespan than their non-gene-mutation-carrying counterparts. A study of Polish breast cancer survivors published in the *Journal of Clinical Oncology* found that when the cancer was caught early, and especially if they underwent the preventive removal of their ovaries (to prevent estrogen from fueling the growth of the breast cancer), their 10-year survival rate was about 80 percent — virtually on par with those survivors not carrying the BRCA1 gene.

These are the clues that a genetic predisposition to breast cancer may exist in your family:

- One or more first-degree relatives, such as your mother or sister, has developed the disease

- Grandmother and mother both developed breast cancer

- Several second-degree relatives, such as grandmothers (but not mothers), aunts, and cousins developed breast cancer

- The relative's cancer occurred in both breasts

- Cancer occurred at a younger-than-average age (This isn't necessarily the case with BRCA1 genetic mutations.)

> **GOOD ADVICE**
>
> If you have breast cancer, get tested to find out if your form was inherited and, if so, inform your siblings and other relatives so they can assess their risk and determine if they should undergo genetic testing.

Stages of Breast Cancer

As with most cancers, the stage at which breast cancer is found predicates its treatment and its prognosis, but it is important to remember that there are survivors at every stage. Staging is also complex, especially in the case of breast cancer, with sub-stage classifications. The precise nature of the staging system illustrates the importance of administering the appropriate course of treatment from the start. Breast cancer staging, like other cancers, takes into account the presence of cancer cells, the size of the tumor (if any), and if/where it has spread.

STAGE 0, OR CANCER IN SITU

In this case, mutated cells are present but have not spread.

- Current guidelines call for a mastectomy for ductal carcinoma in situ. However, some experts believe the treatment to be too radical, and that a lumpectomy or "watchful waiting" are preferable. The 2015 conclusion of a study of 100,000 women over 20 years found a low overall death rate of 3 percent whether a lumpectomy or double mastectomy was performed, making a strong case for less treatment. Of course, other factors like age at diagnosis and genetic predisposition to cancer must be considered.

- **LCIS:** Lobular carcinoma in situ is far less common than DCIS. LCIS rarely becomes cancerous; however, having LCIS is considered a marker for developing cancer in either or both breasts.

STAGE I

This stage indicates that a cancer has formed. Stage I cancers are subdivided into Stages IA and IB. In Stage IA, the tumor is two centimeters or smaller, and no cancer has spread outside the breast. In Stage IB, there may be no cancer, or a cancer two centimeters or smaller, but also tiny clusters of breast cancer cells are present in the lymph nodes.

STAGE II

This stage is divided into two sub-stages:

- **Stage IIA** may be a situation in which no tumor is present in the breast, or there may be a tumor two centimeters or smaller, or cancer larger than two millimeters is found in one to three axillary lymph nodes or in the lymph nodes near the breastbone. Or, the tumor may be between two and five centimeters, but has not spread to the lymph nodes.

- **Stage IIB** describes a tumor between two and five centimeters, with small clusters of breast cancer cells present in the lymph nodes; or the tumor may be the same size as that of Stage IIA, but the cancer has spread to one to three axillary lymph nodes or to the lymph nodes near the breast bone. (Axillary lymph nodes are distributed at the edge of the chest muscles and into the armpits and lower neck.) Or the tumor may be larger than five centimeters, but no cancer has spread to the lymph nodes.

STAGE III

This stage is subdivided into three sub-stages:

- **Stage IIIA** indicates a situation in which a tumor may or may not be present, but cancerous cells have been found in four to nine axillary lymph nodes. Or the tumor may be larger than five centimeters, with cancer found in one to three axillary lymph nodes or lymph nodes near the breastbone.

- **Stage IIIB** breast cancer indicates a tumor of any size, which has spread to the chest wall or to the skin of the breast, causing a swelling or ulcer. Cancer may have spread to the axillary lymph nodes or the lymph nodes near the breastbone.

- **Stage IIIC** may indicate no tumor, or a tumor of any size may have spread to the chest wall and/or the skin of the breast. The cancer has spread to 10 or more axillary lymph nodes; or to the lymph nodes above or below the collarbone; or to axillary lymph nodes and lymph nodes near the breastbone.

STAGE IV
This is a situation in which the cancer has spread to other parts of the body, usually the bones, lungs, liver, or brain.

Signs and Symptoms of Breast Cancer

- **Breast lump:** This is the most common early sign of breast cancer. A lump in the armpit can also signify breast cancer.

- **Change in the size, shape, or feel of the breast or nipple:** Redness, dimpling, or puckering of the breast or nipple may be apparent.

- **Fluid or discharge from the breast or nipple:** Such fluid can be bloody, clear, yellow, or green and pus-like.

- **A red, itchy rash:** This is a sign of inflammatory breast cancer.

Special Diagnostic Tests

Here is a list of tests specifically performed to diagnose breast cancer. To learn more about general cancer testing, see chapter 2.

Clinical Breast Exam
The doctor will perform a physical examination and also examine the breasts for any sign of lumps, changes, or abnormalities. If a

clinical breast exam uncovers an abnormality, one or more of the following imaging tests can be used as a diagnostic second step. They include:

Mammogram

You are probably familiar with mammography as a screening test. A diagnostic mammogram is done to determine if a cancer is present, or to check out other potential breast cancer symptoms, such as breast changes or discharge. A clinical breast exam can also be done in conjunction with mammography.

Other Imaging Tests

Non-invasive ultrasound tests and magnetic resonance imaging (MRI) may be done to provide more information about the breast tumor and also determine if the cancer has spread.

Biopsy or Needle Aspiration

While other tests can suggest the presence of cancer, only a biopsy can confirm the diagnosis. In a biopsy, a small section of tissue is removed and examined under a microscope to see if cancerous cells are present.

Blood Tests and Tumor Markers

If a diagnosis of breast cancer is confirmed, several additional tests are performed. These include examining the tumor for various characteristics and to determine if any proteins, hormones, or other markers are present that can aid in the customization of treatment. For instance, breast cancer receptors are located in the cells of the tumor and the breast, and can influence the type of pharmacological, hormone, or other treatment given. These tests may include the following:

- **Estrogen receptor (ER) and progesterone receptor (PR) tests:** If the tumor has receptors for these hormones, this indicates that they help fuel tumor growth, which is necessary information about how to treat the cancer to prevent a recurrence. About 75 percent to 80 percent of breast cancers have estrogen and/or progesterone receptors.

- **HER2 test:** Breast cancers that show an increase in the number of copies of the HER2 gene (human epidermal growth factor receptor) tend to grow more quickly. This information is absolutely necessary to determine the best treatment. Breast cancers that do not have ER and/or PR receptors or HER2 genes are called "triple-negative" breast cancers. These represent about 15 percent of invasive breast cancers, and are the type that usually grow and spread more quickly. Triple-negative breast cancers are more often found in women with BRCA1 mutations.

- **Genetic testing:** Genetic testing, also known as molecular testing, is another important diagnostic with regard to course of treatment. Via genetic testing, for instance, doctors can learn whether chemotherapy is needed to prevent a cancer recurrence or not. They may also be able to determine whether the cancer cells are more apt to divide quickly and will respond to chemotherapy, or whether they are slower growing and hormone therapy is a better choice.

GOOD ADVICE

You should obtain a copy of your pathology report and have it explained to you in detail. This report contains all of the information that the pathologist observed when looking at cells, including the type, subtype, grade, and stage of your cancer, as well as the characteristics of any hormone receptors that were found. Such information is used to create a treatment plan.

Treatments

When most women think of breast cancer treatment, the term "radical mastectomy" comes to mind. This major form of surgery, which consisted of removing not only the breasts, but also the underlying chest muscles and associated lymph nodes, was the major treatment of breast cancer from 1895 to the mid-1970s, and even beyond. In fact, women would go under anesthesia for a breast biopsy and wake up to find their breasts gone. Such traumatic experiences have haunted generations of women.

Fortunately, clinical trials have finally proven that, in the case of breast cancer surgery, "more" is not necessarily better. "We used to over-treat breast cancer like crazy, but now we have much more of a handle on what treatment is appropriate, so our treatment is more targeted with less side effects," says Dr. Link.

The importance of conservative treatment, or doing the least amount of surgery that will be effective, pertains not only to the breasts, but also to the lymph nodes. Lymph nodes are small structures that filter out harmful substances. They are arranged in a network of vessels and are the primary way that breast cancer spreads to other parts of the body. Until recently, clinical guidelines advised complete axillary node removal of all 20 to 30 lymph nodes if a woman's sentinel biopsy was positive, no matter whether other lymph nodes were suspicious or not. (The sentinel node describes the first node to which the cancer is likely to spread.) Recently, though, a study in the *Journal of the American Medical Association* found that the results were just as good for women who had only the sentinel node removed, as opposed to the other nodes as well, as long as they were not affected. This is important, because the removal of lymph nodes can cause shoulder and arm symptoms including lymphedema, severe pain or numbness, and reduced range of motion.

Types of Surgery
MASTECTOMY

A mastectomy is the removal of one or two breasts. Although one or both breasts are removed, this surgery is less disfiguring than the radical mastectomy, with fewer side effects and quicker recovery. Mastectomies are done for the following reasons:

- DCIS
- Stage I and II breast cancer
- Locally advanced cancer (Stage III)
- Inflammatory breast cancer
- Paget disease of the breast

Women who have a mastectomy may wish to consider breast reconstruction, which is surgery to create a breast substitute. Reconstruction may be done with tissue from another part of the body or with synthetic implants. Reconstruction can be done at the same time as the mastectomy (immediate reconstruction) or at some point in the future (delayed reconstruction). This decision may depend on the characteristics of the particular cancer.

BREAST CONSERVING SURGERY

This form of surgery has replaced the radical mastectomy. Known also as **local control**, it allows for the removal of the cancer while leaving the breast in place.

The two major types of breast conserving surgery are lumpectomy, known also as **wide local excision**, or a partial mastectomy. For either to be performed, the cancer must be in the form of a small single tumor that can be removed completely. These surgeries are followed by radiation, which itself poses a risk of cancer and therefore is administered extremely conservatively, so the woman must never have undergone it before. A partial mastectomy is similar to a lumpectomy, but the size of the tumor can be larger.

Women who undergo a lumpectomy or partial mastectomy may consider a type of reconstruction known as **oncoplastic surgery**, which is done to match the breasts.

MASTECTOMY VS. LUMPECTOMY

Women with early-stage breast cancer will often receive a choice of whether to undergo a lumpectomy or opt for a mastectomy. On the surface, this choice might seem obvious, with most women opting to retain their breasts, but the choice is actually more complicated, Dr. Link says.

"There has been a huge increase of young women under age 40, 45, or 50 getting bilateral mastectomies who, in the past, would have gotten a lumpectomy with radiation. Part of this is due to the phenomenal results of plastic surgery with skin and nipple sparing. A lot of them are doing it because they don't want to risk the cancer recurring, or they don't want to go for periodic MRIs and biopsies."

Because of such options, it's best to take your time to make your decision. Seek out a second opinion, or even a third, so you're confident you've made the right choice.

Other Modes of Therapy

CHEMOTHERAPY

Neoadjuvant chemotherapy is administered before surgery and is usually done to shrink early-stage breast cancer tumors so they can be removed during local, breast-sparing surgery. **Adjuvant chemotherapy** is administered after surgery. This is given to prevent the cancer from recurring. Chemotherapy is also used for cancers that have metastasized, or spread.

There is now an enormous array of chemotherapy drugs available, specific to the treatment of a variety of types of breast cancer. Research has also shown that certain drugs are more effective when given in combination, especially for adjuvant therapy.

IMMUNOTHERAPY

As opposed to chemotherapy, immunotherapy agents work by interfering with specific molecules to block the growth and spread of cancer. Such available agents for HER2-positive cancers are **trastuzumab, pertuzmab**, and **lapitinib**, though this is still an active research area.

HORMONAL THERAPY

This type of therapy is used to treat most tumors that test positive for either estrogen or progesterone receptors. The drugs effectively treat certain tumors by blocking the tumor's receptors, cutting off the cancer cells' fuel source, causing them to die. Tamoxifen, which blocks estrogen receptors, has proven revolutionary, not only in lowering the risk of recurrence in women who have had cancer, but also in preventing cancer in those at high risk of developing the disease.

Another type of hormonal therapy is the use of **aromatase inhibitors (AIs)**. These decrease the amount of estrogen made by tissues other than the ovaries in postmenopausal women by blocking the aromatase enzyme. This enzyme changes weak male hormones, called androgens, into estrogen when the ovaries have stopped making estrogen during menopause. These drugs include **anastrozole (Arimidex)**, **letrozole (Femara)**, and **exemestane (Aromasin)**.

RADIATION

Radiation therapy is typically given after a lumpectomy, and also following adjuvant chemotherapy, if recommended. In fact, modern surgery and radiation therapy are credited with reducing the risk that breast cancer will recur to less than five percent over the 10 years after treatment. This is the case whether the surgery was a lumpectomy or a mastectomy.

Adjuvant radiation therapy is also recommended for some women after a mastectomy. Whether or not radiation is warranted depends on the patient's age, the size of the tumor, the number of lymph nodes found to contain cancer, whether the tumor was removed cleanly (clear margins), whether the tumor is hormone sensitive, if it is HER2 status, and other factors.

Breast Cancer in Men

Robert Kaitz was a busy 53-year-old entrepreneur when he saw his doctor in 2006 for what he figured would be a simple office visit for a sore throat. Almost as an afterthought, he told the doctor he had a lump behind his nipple. "I figured it was a cyst, but the doctor told me you don't get cysts there," Kaitz recalls.

The diagnosis turned out to be advanced breast cancer, and within weeks, he was undergoing treatment. "I'm known for my sense of humor, so when people would ask, 'What kind of cancer do you have?' and I'd answer, 'breast cancer,' they'd pause and wait for the joke."

There was no punch line — Kaitz indeed had breast cancer, and because the lump had been there for well over a year, the cancer had plenty of time to spread. As a result, he had to undergo a radical mastectomy, two rounds of chemotherapy and two rounds of radiation, before he was declared cancer-free.

"I was absolutely fortunate, but if I knew that men could get breast cancer, I would have gone to the doctor much sooner," says Kaitz, especially since his mother is a breast cancer survivor. But, like most people, he simply assumed that men don't develop breast cancer. Through rare, breast cancer more commonly occurs in men between 60 and 70 years old, but it may occur at any age.

"Some cancers are caught early, and the men do extremely well. If the cancer is caught later, it's more difficult. It's like any other breast cancer," says Neil B. Friedman, MD, a breast cancer surgeon and director of the Hoffberger Breast Center at Mercy Medical Center in Baltimore, Maryland.

A recent study on breast cancer in men confirmed that survival rates are lower because their cancers tend to be diagnosed at a

DID YOU KNOW . . .

Chemotherapy was once automatically administered following breast cancer surgery, but this is no longer the case because of the increased understanding of breast cancer, and the knowledge that some tumors respond to chemotherapy and some do not. Now, whether a woman should undergo chemotherapy is decided on a case-by-case basis.

more advanced stage. And, as with women, the biggest known risk factor is genetic — BRCA 1 and BRCA 2 genes play the very same role in both genders.

Here are the other risk factors for breast cancer in men:

- Gynecomastia — abnormal enlargement of the breast
- Radiation exposure to the chest
- Estrogen exposure (during prostate cancer treatment, for instance)
- Obesity
- Severe liver disease
- Klinefelter syndrome, a rare genetic condition

Breast cancer in men is treated generally the same as it is in women. Depending on the stage of the cancer, surgery and/or chemotherapy or radiation may be needed. Hormone therapy, especially the drug **tamoxifen**, is also used to treat male breast cancer.

Lung Cancer

7

JENNY WHITE WAS CLEANING her bathroom when she unwittingly breathed in a noxious combination of bleach and bathroom cleaner that sent her into a coughing fit and eventually to see her doctor. He sent her for a chest X-ray, which showed an unrelated nodule on her lung. Her doctor monitored it and, since it was growing, she had no choice but to undergo surgery so a biopsy could be taken.

"My doctor had told me before the surgery that if I saw one chest tube in me when I awakened, it meant that the nodule was harmless, but if I saw two, it was cancer. When I awoke, I saw the two tubes," she recalls. Stunned, Jenny, a lifelong smoker, realized she was dealing with lung cancer.

What Is Lung Cancer?

Also known as pulmonary carcinoma, lung cancer forms just like other cancers — abnormal cells begin to grow and divide at an uncontrollable rate. In the case of the lungs, the two sponge-like organs that make up the main component of the respiratory system, cancerous cells form a tumor, lesion, or nodule. As cells continue to multiply, nearby tissues and organs are also threatened by the disease.

When we breathe, our lungs drink in oxygen, and when we exhale, they expel carbon dioxide, the waste product our body's cells produce. This process is vital for life. As the cancer grows and spreads, it becomes impossible for the lungs to serve this very important, life-giving function.

Statistics

There are about 250,000 new cases of lung cancer each year, roughly affecting men and women equally, and resulting in an estimated 160,000 deaths each year, which accounts for about 27 percent of all cancer deaths.

Lung cancer is by far the leading cause of cancer death among both men and women. Each year, more people die of lung cancer than of colon, breast, and prostate cancers combined. Traditionally thought of as a man's disease, it is now an equal opportunity killer. This is because lung cancer may take up to 20 years to develop, and women historically began smoking heavily about two decades or so after men.

"The incidence of lung cancer has decreased slightly in men because a lot of men who used to smoke quit, but not in women because they started smoking later," says Bruno Bastos, MD, an oncologist who specializes in lung cancer at Cleveland Clinic Florida.

Lung cancer mainly occurs in older people. About two-thirds of those diagnosed with lung cancer are 65 or older; fewer than two percent of all cases are found in people younger than 45. The average age at the time of diagnosis is about 70.

Overall, the chance that a man will develop lung cancer in his lifetime is about one in 13; for a woman, the risk is about one in 16. (These numbers include both smokers and non-smokers.)

Outcome and Survival Rates

There are about 400,000 lung cancer survivors living in the United States today. "Although the survival rate for lung cancer has stayed relatively unchanged, it is expected to climb thanks to new treatments. In the meantime, the quality of life for lung cancer patients is improving," Dr. Bastos says.

If lung cancer is caught at its earliest stage (Stage 0), the survival rate is 60 to 80 percent. If it is caught at Stage I or Stage II, the survival rate is 40 to 50 percent. For people with large tumors, but no evidence of spread, this may be higher. The survival rate for Stage III lung cancer is about 23 percent, and if the cancer reaches Stage IV, this figure drops to 10 percent.

It is important to recognize, though, that lung cancer can be diagnosed at any of the stages. In addition, the type, size, and location of the cancer can make a big difference. Typically, women survive with lung cancer longer than do men. Whether or not other lung diseases are present also makes a difference.

SMOKING AND LUNG CANCER

It will come as no shock that the chief cause of lung cancer is cigarette smoking. Although people who are non-smokers can get lung cancer, well over 80 percent of cases are due to smoking. People who smoke cigars, pipes, and even marijuana are also at higher risk, although not as high as those who smoke cigarettes.

Cigarette smoke contains thousands of chemical compounds, many of which are carcinogenic (cancer-causing). When we smoke, our lungs retain 70 to 90 percent of these compounds. There is also is evidence that these chemicals damage DNA, the body's genetic code, paving the way for cancer to develop.

How much do you need to smoke to develop cancer? Experts discuss this question in terms of "pack-years." They place at highest risk the smoker who has accumulated 30 pack-years. This amount can be accrued in different ways: a person can smoke a pack a day for 30 years, two packs for 15 years, three packs for 10 years, and so on.

But don't confuse these distinctions with real life. In real life, there's no magic number; susceptibility to cancer varies widely from person to person. Some people can smoke their entire, long lives and remain cancer-free; others may never have smoked even one cigarette and develop the disease.

Not all smokers get lung cancer, which is an indication that genetics is involved. People with relatives who developed lung cancer are at higher risk than others. In addition, chronic obstructive pulmonary disease, or COPD (the umbrella label for a group of diseases that include emphysema and chronic bronchitis), increases lung cancer risk.

"Although smoking is by far the greatest risk factor, some non-smokers do develop lung cancer. This is true of both men and women non-smokers, but there appears to be an albeit small, but growing group comprised of female lung cancer victims who have developed the disease for, thus far, no explicable reason," says Dr. Bastos. Indeed, statistics show that one in five women who develop lung cancer are non-smokers.

Although cigarette smoke accounts for the vast majority of lung cancer cases, a host of environmental pollutants can play a role. Chief among these is asbestos, a carcinogenic material used mainly for things like insulation and brake linings. Over the years, the awareness of the danger posed by asbestos has grown and we've limited our exposure. Asbestos is still found in some places, although removing it — causing fibers to become airborne — sometimes poses more of a danger than leaving it in place. Lung cancer from exposure to asbestos can take decades to develop.

Radon is another lung cancer risk factor. This radioactive gas, which is given off by uranium, thorium, certain rocks, and soil, surrounds us. In open areas, radon diffuses into the air, so low-level, outdoor exposure is not harmful, but it can seep into buildings, such as homes, as well. Large concentrations of radon in poorly ventilated conditions (like underground mines), pose an extremely detrimental threat.

Long-term exposure to air pollution also heightens risk because it is filled with some of the same toxic gases, such as nitrogen oxide and carbon monoxide, found in cigarette smoke.

In addition, excessive alcohol use (more than three drinks a day) is associated with higher lung cancer risk. Since many people are inclined to smoke while imbibing alcoholic drinks, this would obviously raise the risk more.

Some diseases — or the treatment for them — will hike lung cancer risk as well. For example, radiation to treat breast cancer or blood cancers (like leukemia and non-Hodgkin's lymphoma), raises the risk, even decades later.

Types of Lung Cancer

There are many different forms of pulmonary carcinoma, but the more common ones are broadly divided into two basic categories: small cell lung cancer and non-small cell lung cancer.

SMALL CELL CARCINOMA

This is the more aggressive, but less common type of lung cancer. Its small, oat-like cells (which is why it's also known as oat-cell cancer) occur in the tissue of the lungs and often it is not diagnosed until it has spread elsewhere in the body. It is usually found in smokers and former smokers. This type of carcinoma accounts for 15 to 20 percent of all cases.

GOOD ADVICE

US military personnel who were exposed to Agent Orange during the Vietnam War are vulnerable to lung cancer. If you are a Vietnam veteran, you should qualify for a VA Disability compensation and special access to medical care. You do not need to prove that your exposure to Agent Orange caused your cancer. See the appendix for more information.

NON-SMALL CELL LUNG CANCER (NSCLC)

This type of lung cancer grows more slowly than small cell carcinoma. Non-small cell is the largest category of lung cancer and accounts for some 80 percent of lung cancer cases.

Although there are other, rarer types of non-small cell lung cancers, this form of pulmonary carcinoma is divided into major three types:

- **Squamous cell:** Also called epidermoid, this type of cancer begins in the lung's central areas or in one of the two major air passages and grows slowly. It occurs more commonly in men. Epidermoid lung cancers are almost always caused by smoking.

- **Adenocarcinoma:** This type often develops along the outer edges of the lung and under the membranes of the large air passages of the lungs. It is the most common type of lung cancer, and slightly more predominant in women.

- **Large cell lung cancer:** Large, abnormal cells characterize this type of lung cancer, which usually begins in the smaller breathing tubes, but can appear anywhere in the lungs.

Stages of Lung Cancer

STAGE 0, OR CARCINOMA IN SITU

This describes abnormal cells that have not grown beyond the lining of the airways. Again, if the cancer is described as being in situ, this means that it is non-invasive, and, at this early stage, is not yet capable of spreading to other regions. As the cancer grows, however, it may spread. Lung cancer that is caught this early is usually picked up accidentally, possibly due to a person getting a chest X-ray or CT scan for some other reason.

STAGE I

This stage involves a situation in which the cancer is confined to the lung and hasn't spread to the lymph nodes. The tumor is generally three centimeters or smaller.

STAGE II

This describes a tumor that is not larger than seven centimeters and may have spread to areas nearby, such as the chest wall, the diaphragm, the lining around the lungs or heart, or the area not less than two centimeters below where the trachea meets the bronchus (the large airway that bridges the trachea and lung). The cancer may also have spread to the nearby lymph nodes. The portion of the lung where the trachea meets the bronchus may be collapsed or inflamed. One lobe of the lung may contain one or more separate tumors.

STAGE III

This stage is marked by the cancer's invasion of other organs near the lungs, like the heart and its major blood vessels, the esophagus, and larynx (voice box). The tumor(s) may be large, but even in the event of smaller tumors, cancer cells may be present in the lymph nodes farther away from the lungs. Part of the lung may have collapsed or become inflamed.

STAGE IV

The cancer has spread beyond the affected lung to the other lung and to distant areas of the body, such as the brain, liver, kidneys, or bones.

Signs and Symptoms of Lung Cancer

Lung cancer is so dangerous because it usually causes no early symptoms, which provides it with the opportunity to spread before it is diagnosed. If lung cancer develops in the windpipe, it does cause a cough, but too often that is brushed off as "smoker's cough." It is important to bring any of these symptoms to a doctor's attention immediately:

- Persistent, deep, wheezing cough

- Increased sputum (mucus) which may be streaked with blood

- Chronic chest pain

- Belabored breathing

- Recurring pneumonia or bronchitis

- Difficulty swallowing

- Hoarseness

- Arm and shoulder pain (this can occur in one type of rare lung cancer)

- Fatigue

Lung Cancer Screening

For the past several years, researchers have been testing low-dose, spiral CAT screening to determine whether the method could be used for early detection of lung cancer. Finally, in 2013, enough evidence had been collected proving that, for high-risk individuals, the benefits of this type of screening greatly outweigh

DID YOU KNOW . . .

Fatigue can be a common warning sign of lung cancer. Unfortunately, this symptom is also easily overlooked or misinterpreted as a normal sign of aging, or of a common ailment, like the flu.

the dangers (complications from low-dose radiation exposure). The US Preventive Services Task Force now recommends that current smokers between the ages of 55 and 80 or those who have quit within the past 15 years undergo screening. The task force defines high-risk as those who have 30 pack-years or more.

Specific Diagnostic Tests

PHYSICAL EXAMINATION

The doctor will take a detailed inventory of the patient's symptoms, medical history, and smoking history, and will also perform a general examination.

SPUTUM CYTOLOGY

A sample of mucus will be taken and examined under a microscope to look for signs of cancer. The doctor will collect a sample by having the patient cough (often induced by having the patient breathe a saline mist) or via a **bronchoscopy** — a procedure that enables the doctor to insert a scope in order to view the patient's airways, at which time a sample may be taken as well.

CHEST X-RAY

Not suitable for early lung cancer screening, chest X-rays are able to pick up more advanced tumors. Smaller tumors will not show up on chest X-rays, necessitating a CT (or CAT) scan or other imaging test.

CT SCAN (ALSO CALLED A CAT, SPIRAL CT, OR HELICAL SCAN)

This more sophisticated imaging test can detect smaller tumors, making it a far more reliable tool than a chest X-ray for detecting lung cancer in its earlier stages. The CT scan is the best method available for lung cancer screening; however, since it exposes the recipient to low doses of radiation, the test is recommended only to those who are considered high-risk for the disease (current or former smokers between 55 and 74 with a 30 pack-year or more history).

OTHER IMAGING TESTS

These include magnetic resonance imaging (MRI) and positron emission tomography (PET scan), which are done both to detect tumors and to see if they have spread.

BIOPSY

In order to confirm the diagnosis of lung cancer as well as determine the cell type to correctly recommend treatment, this test must be performed. A biopsy involves removing a bit of tissue from the lungs and examining it under a microscope. A biopsy is also performed to determine the stage of the cancer.

BRONCHOSCOPY

The doctor uses a thin viewing instrument, the bronchoscope, to view the airway, lungs, or lymph nodes of the chest to check for signs of cancer. A bronchoscopy can also be done to remove tissue samples for biopsy.

MEDIASTINOSCOPY

This is a surgical procedure that calls for the making of a small cut in the neck or on the left side of the chest. Then a thin scope called a mediastinoscope is inserted through the opening in order to explore the mediastinum (the space between the lungs). This is another way to perform a biopsy.

PULMONARY FUNCTION TEST

An evaluation of lung capacity is measured, either by means of breathing tests or by having the patient inhale nitrogen or helium for a specific period of time, after which the amount of gas in the lungs is measured to determine lung volume.

THORACENTESIS

The doctor will insert a needle between the lung and the chest wall, collecting fluid to be checked for cancer cells.

THORACOSCOPY

An endoscope (a thin, tubelike instrument outfitted with a camera) is placed into an incision made in the skin to examine the pleura (membrane lining chest cavity and the outside of each lung), lungs, and mediastinum, and also remove tissue for examination.

BLOOD TESTS AND TUMOR MARKERS

Lung cancer can secrete proteins and hormones into the bloodstream. These tumor markers can furnish important information as to the diagnosis, type of tumor, and evaluating what types of treatments might be most effective.

Such molecular testing is not being done often enough. In fact, a 2015 study showed that 25 percent of patients who might have benefited from such testing missed out. So a consortium of organizations has come out with guidelines specifying that all patients with advanced lung adenocarcinoma should be tested for abnormalities in two genes: EGFR and ALK. Patients with the EGFR abnormality can be treated with **Tarceva (erlotinib)**, and those with ALK can receive **Xalkori (crizotinib)**. In addition, clinical testing is underway for new drugs targeting these genetic abnormalities.

> **GOOD ADVICE**
>
> Before any type of treatment is initiated, make sure that your biopsy report is read by a pathologist with experience in lung cancer diagnosis and that you receive a copy of the report. According to Dr. Bastos, "Today, it's not acceptable to receive a report that says that you have non-small cell cancer. The pathologist must also stipulate the specific type of cancer. For instance, if you have non-small cell lung cancer, the report should say if it is adenocarcinoma, squamous cell carcinoma, large cell carcinoma, or a more rare form."

Treatments

There are four types of treatments for lung cancer: surgery, chemotherapy, radiation therapy, and targeted therapy. The treatment depends on the type of cancer found and whether it has spread to the lymph nodes and/or to other parts of the body.

SURGERY

Small cell lung cancer is very aggressive, fast-growing, and very often has extensively spread by the time it is discovered. Therefore, surgery is only curative in a very small number of patients (about five percent). However, when surgery is done on these patients in combination with chemotherapy and radiation, it can result in a 35 to 40 percent cure rate.

Non-small cell lung cancer grows more slowly, so the chance of discovering it while the tumor is still operable is greater.

CHEMOTHERAPY

Chemical treatment may be administered before surgery to try and shrink the tumor, after surgery to keep the cancer from returning, or as the main type of treatment in lung cancer cases that are too far advanced for surgery.

RADIATION

Radiation can be used as the main treatment for tumors that cannot be surgically removed. Radiation can also be done to shrink the tumor before surgery or afterwards to kill any remaining cancer cells and prevent recurrence.

There are several different types of radiation that can be used for lung cancer, including high-dose brachytherapy (also called high-dose remote radiation), which is used on people with lung cancers located in the major bronchi, or breathing passages.

IMMUNOTHERAPY

This personalized medicine requires genetic testing on tumors to determine if they can be treated with drugs targeted specifically for them. **Opdivo (nivolumab)**, FDA approved in 2015, is the first immunotherapy drug for non-small cell lung cancer. In a clinical trial, it extended the lifespan of 30 percent of patients by two years.

Jenny White, whose story was told at the beginning of this chapter, credits this type of therapy with helping save her life. "Because I had cancer, my surgeon sent me to an oncologist after my surgery who suggested I have my tumor tested for a biomarker. It turned out to be positive for the EGFR mutation, which is more common in non-smokers, so I underwent chemotherapy targeted at that. My oncologist said that before that, I had an 85 percent chance of survival, but this would squash any rogue cells and get that estimate up to 95 percent," she says.

What Happens If Lung Cancer Spreads?

One of the areas that lung cancer tends to spread, especially in women, is to the brain. While this is obviously not good, it does not mean that the situation is hopeless, says Lee M. Tessler, MD, a neurosurgeon and executive

GOOD ADVICE

"Lung cancer patients often think that quitting smoking [once they're diagnosed] is 'closing the barn door after the horse is out,' but this is not true. Quitting smoking is the most important thing lung cancer patients can do to boost their chance of survival," says Dr. Bastos.

director of the Long Island Brain Tumor Center. "Once, if lung cancer spread to the brain, that was it. But now, we can use [new] techniques to treat it, and so people are living for years, even though their cancers had spread to the brain," he says. And, he adds, "their quality of life is good too" — a message he is trying to bring not only to patients, but to their oncologists as well. See the chapter on brain cancer for a list of treatment techniques.

8

Colon Cancer

JUAN FLOREZ WAS 61 when he went for a routine physical and his doctor told him he was anemic. He had no other symptoms, but his doctor suggested he undergo a colonoscopy. His doctor had been suggesting the test for a year, but the retired postmaster had brushed him off. Now, though, there was no choice. Immediately after the test was over, the doctor returned. "He told me, 'You have cancer and it needs to come out,'" Florez recalls.

Because his cancer had spread, Florez had to undergo not only surgery, but also nine months of chemotherapy, from which he still suffers some nerve damage. But now, five years later, he feels extremely lucky: "It was Stage IV cancer and I know many people do not beat that, so I feel very fortunate to have beaten those odds," he says.

What Is Colon Cancer?

The colon is part of the large intestine, and is one of the organs of the digestive system that deals with waste. Since the colon is attached to the rectum, colon cancer sometimes goes by the term **colorectal cancer**, which encompasses cancer that occurs in the colon or in the rectum.

The colon is particularly vulnerable to turning cancerous because the organ's cells are constantly growing and dividing, and also because the cells come into contact with digested food by-products that can be carcinogenic (cancer-promoting). Colon cancer arises from polyps, which are a precancerous type of growth that forms on the lining of the colon.

This chapter focuses primarily on colon cancer. Rectal cancer, while similar, is treated slightly differently, as is noted later in this chapter.

Statistics

There are well over one million colon cancer survivors living in the United States today (roughly 600,000 men and 600,000 women). An estimated 145,000 people will be diagnosed this year, and about 50,000 people will lose their battle with the disease. Colon cancer is the third most common cancer and the second leading cause of death (after lung cancer) for men and women combined.

Generally, one in every 20 Americans risks developing colon cancer, and that risk increases with age. Only three percent of colon cancers arise in those younger than 40. Generally, the risk of colon cancer begins to mount after the age of 55, and 80 percent of all colon cancer occurs in people over the age of 65; however, if colon cancer runs in your family, you are at risk at a much younger age.

Colon cancer can occur in people without risk factors, but there is a connection to genetics; having a family history of colon cancer raises risk, even if direct heredity is not involved.

"Whenever a patient is diagnosed with colon cancer, we take a very detailed family history. We also test the tumor and look for specific genetic mutations, because we want to alert the family," says Dr. Juan Nogueras, who is a colorectal surgeon at the Cleveland Clinic Florida.

"Even if this is the first time colon cancer has occurred in a family, if there is a certain mutation, it could have the potential of being passed down to the patient's children," Dr. Nogueras notes.

Familial adenomatous polyposis (FAP) is an inherited form of colon cancer that results in people as young as 30 developing carpets of polyps on the walls of the colon. Lynch syndrome is another type of genetically inherited colon cancer. One type of **Lynch syndrome**, also known as **hereditary non-polyposis colorectal cancer**, or **HNPCC**, can cause a smaller number of polyps, and another type heightens the risk of not only colon cancer, but also uterine (or endometrial cancer), ovarian and, less commonly, bladder cancer as well.

There is a difference between having a strong family history and those whose family history puts them at less risk, but still higher than average risk. A person with a parent, brother, or sister who developed colon cancer at an earlier-than-expected age (about 55) is at higher risk than those who have relatives with colon cancer clustered on one side of the family, such as aunts, uncles, cousins, or grandparents, but not a parent. They are still at higher risk, though.

Having had colon or rectal polyps in the past indicates an increased risk of colon cancer. Chronic inflammatory bowel disease, which includes ulcerative colitis and Crohn's disease, increases the risk of colon cancer; however, the common stomach malady known as irritable bowel syndrome does not.

Obesity increases the risk of colon cancer, and there are conflicting studies that link a traditional high-fat low-fiber, American diet to colon cancer. As with many other cancers, smoking also increases the risk of colon cancer.

GOOD ADVICE

If you are diagnosed with colon cancer, you should make your family members aware of it as they might want to consider undergoing genetic screening and/or regular colon cancer screening as well.

Outcome and Survival Rates

The colon cancer death rate is declining, probably due to early detection because, like other types of cancer, the survival rate declines once the cancerous cells spread to other organs.

If the cancer is diagnosed in its earliest stage, the five-year survival rate is 90 percent. If it has spread to nearby lymph nodes and organs, that number dips to 70 percent. If the cancer has spread to distant organs, the survival rate declines to 12 percent. However, in the case of colon cancer, its stage doesn't tell the whole story.

According to national registry data, some third-stage colon cancer sufferers can have a better survival rate than that of second stage; it all depends on the particular case. For instance, if colon cancer spreads and results in only one or a few tumors in the lungs or liver, surgery may be able to remove them, resulting in a higher chance of a cure.

Types of Colon Cancer

Most colon cancers are a type of tumor called adenocarcinoma, which arise from the inside tissue of the colon and rectum. This chapter focuses on this type of tumor. Other types of cancer that occur far less often but can begin in the colon or rectum include **carcinoid tumor**, **gastrointestinal stromal tumor (GIST)**, and **lymphoma**.

Stages of Colon Cancer

As with other forms of cancer, the stage at which it is diagnosed determines both the patient's prognosis and treatment.

STAGE 0, OR CARCINOMA IN SITU

This describes a situation in which cancerous cells are found only in the innermost lining **(mucosa)** of the colon.

STAGE I

The cancer has spread beyond the mucosa to the second and third layers of the inside of the colon — the **submucosa** and the **muscle wall**.

STAGE II

Tumors are larger and extend through the mucosa, submucosa, and muscular wall of the colon to the outermost layer of the colon **(serosa)**, but the cancer has not spread to the lymph nodes.

STAGE III

Tumors have spread through the serosa (outside the colon) to one or more of the lymph nodes, and the cure rate has dropped to 65 percent.

STAGE IV

The cancer has spread outside the colon and through the lymph nodes to other parts of the body, such as the liver, lungs, or in women, the ovaries, and survival rate has dropped to about 10 percent.

Signs and Symptoms

- Changes in bowel habits, such as constipation and diarrhea
- Very dark, mahogany-red, or bright-red blood in or on the stool

- Abdominal discomfort

- Persistent narrowing of the stools

- Urgent, painful need to defecate

- Feeling that you cannot completely empty your bowel

- Anemia

- Unexplained weight loss

- Unusual paleness

- Fatigue

The most common symptom of [colorectal] cancer is bleeding from the rectum," says Dr. Nogueras. Other symptoms, however, can vary and also may depend on where the tumor is located. "If the cancer is located on the left side of the colon, there are more symptoms of blockage, such as changes in the bowels and bleeding. If the tumor is on the right side, then an earlier sign can be anemia because there is a loss of blood due to the tumor."

The abdominal symptoms of colon cancer mimic such non-cancerous disorders as irritable bowel syndrome and ulcerative colitis, or even the flu. But if you don't have one of these disorders and you suddenly begin suffering these symptoms, give it a few days. If the symptoms disappear, it may have been the flu. If not, make an appointment with your doctor or healthcare provider.

Colon Cancer Screening

Colon cancer is slow-growing. There are recommended screening tests that can be performed to detect it while it is still in its earliest, most treatable stage. The tests and schedule for screening are as follows:

- **Colonoscopy:** Once every 10 years

- **Flexible sigmoidoscopy:** One every five years, or, if combined with a fecal occult blood test, every three years

- **Fecal occult blood test:** Every year

DID YOU KNOW . . .

Most people think that blood in the stool will turn out to be bright red, but that isn't necessarily true. In many cases, the stool may turn the color of rust or brick-red instead.

The Centers for Disease Control guidelines call for all adults between the ages of 50 and 75 to be screened using one of these three tests. But according to the latest statistics, an estimated one-third of Americans are not being screened. Government health officials believe this is partly because the screening test that is most often recommended, the colonoscopy, is considered uncomfortable, expensive, and can require a day off from work. (The flexible sigmoidoscopy also carries the same drawbacks as a colonoscopy.) But although a colonoscopy is the best screening test, there is another option that is easier and that people might be more willing to do, and this is the fecal occult blood test (FOBT).

This stool test does not test for cancer, but for the presence of blood in the stool. It requires you to put a tiny dab of stool onto a special card for processing. Then, when a chemical is applied, the stool changes in color if blood is present. This is blood that is invisible to the naked eye, but its presence can present an early cancer warning sign. It's important to note, though, that the presence of blood does not necessarily indicate cancer; many noncancerous conditions can cause it as well, such as hemorrhoids. Also, this test is not as foolproof as a colonoscopy, because some tumors bleed only intermittently and some do not bleed at all.

So, if you are one of those people who do not want to undergo a colonoscopy or a flexible sigmoidoscopy for screening, you should opt for an annual stool test as an easy way to screen for colorectal cancer. As Tom Frieden, the head of the CDC, has noted, "The best test is the test that gets done."

Specific Diagnostic Tests
DIGITAL RECTAL EXAM
The doctor inserts a gloved finger into your rectum. This is the most common test to check for colorectal cancer, and it can detect a small number of them, but it is actually more effective at finding prostate cancer in men.

COLONOSCOPY
The doctor uses an instrument called a colonoscope, which can view the entire colon. This is the main diagnostic test for colon cancer today.

BARIUM ENEMA
This can be an alternative to a colonoscopy. For this, a tube with barium is passed into the intestine and X-rays are taken. It should

be noted, however, that although the barium enema is less expensive than a colonoscopy, it doesn't visualize abnormalities with as much clarity as a colonoscopy does.

BIOPSY

A small amount of tissue is removed from the colon for testing. Sometimes, a CT scan or ultrasound helps the surgeon guide the needle into the tumor for tissue removal.

BLOOD TESTS AND TUMOR MARKERS

Colon cancer cells can secrete proteins known as tumor markers. Identifying and monitoring them can help your oncologist customize your treatment. In the case of colon cancer, tests will show if the tumor is a candidate for treatment with **panitumumab (Vectibix)**, a monoclonal antibody that attaches to **EGFRs (epidermal growth factor receptors)** and prevents them from sending growth signals.

IMAGING TESTS

Chest X-rays, CT or CAT scans, PET scans, and bone scans are among the tests that can be used to see if the cancer has spread.

Treatments

Surgery to remove colon cancer plays a huge role in Stages 0 and 1. That's when the cancer is usually completely removable and no further treatment is needed. For Stage II, surgery may be the only treatment, although chemotherapy may be given to guard against recurrence. Stage III generally requires surgery and removal of all lymph nodes involved, followed by chemotherapy.

TYPES OF SURGERY

Polypectomy: One or more polyps removed during colonoscopy.

- **Local Incision:** The cancer and nearby tissue is removed from the rectal wall through the anus or small cut in the rectum.

- **Colectomy:** The removal of all or part of the colon. The remaining sections are reconnected, sometimes with a new escape route in the abdomen for waste. The opening, called a stoma, is fitted with a pouching system for waste collection.

- **Laparoscopy:** A minimally invasive surgery using a fiberoptic instrument fed through a very small incision.

Radiation also may be needed, depending on the size and aggressiveness of the cancer. Surgery is also the general protocol for Stage IV colon cancer in order to remove the colon or other organs where the cancer may have spread, along with chemotherapy. Radiation is often needed as well. There is also a very aggressive, controversial treatment known as **hyperthermic intraperitoneal chemotherapy**, or **HIPEC**, which may hold promise for carefully selected patients with advanced colon cancer. See chapter 3 for details.

Prostate Cancer

9

HALL OF FAME SPORTS writer Jack McCallum learned he had cancer just in the same way as many other men — undergoing an annual prostate screening test, known as a PSA. "Your PSA is 3.8. That's not overly high, but the concern is how it has steadily risen," he recalls his doctor saying.

McCallum wasn't alarmed, but he was concerned. Cancer was on his radar. He had brushed aside any suggestions from his doctor that he submit to an annual cardiac stress test because he was convinced that, due to his family's medical history, when it was his time to go, "the Big C" would get him, not heart disease.

Still, he was unprepared to learn he had early stage prostate cancer. His story ended well, and he is now cancer-free after surgery, but the experience sent him on an emotional rollercoaster ride fraught with difficult decisions, fear, and uncertainty — so much so that this life-altering journey inspired him to write a book about it. *The Prostate Monologues* focuses on how much is still unknown about this disease, and the ramifications it poses for the men who face it.

What Is Prostate Cancer?

The prostate gland, exclusive to men, is an exocrine gland of the reproductive system. It secretes the majority of what constitutes semen and aids in the ejaculatory process. In order for the gland to function properly, it requires testosterone.

A soft gland a bit larger than the size of a walnut, it is located behind the penis, below the bladder, and in front of the rectum (thus, it can be felt during a rectal exam). The prostate surrounds the urethra at the neck of the bladder.

Made up of various types of cells, it is primarily the glandular cells of the prostate that become cancerous. (These are the cells responsible for the secretion that becomes part of seminal fluid.) Glandular prostate cancer is known as adenocarcinoma. While most adenocarcinomas grow slowly and remain confined to the prostate, some can grow and spread quite rapidly. Though other cancers, like sarcomas and small cell carcinomas do occur, they are extremely rare.

Statistics

About 240,000 men are diagnosed with prostate cancer each year, making it the most common cancer that occurs in men. The median age at diagnosis is 67, and about 30,000 deaths will occur annually due to the disease.

The greatest risk factor for prostate cancer is age. Risk begins to climb after the age of 50, and more than 80 percent of prostate cancers are diagnosed in men who are 65 or older. African-American men are at higher risk than Caucasian men, and Hispanic men are at lower risk, but men of all ethnicities can develop the disease.

About 75 percent of all prostate cancers are sporadic, which means they occur for no known reason. Although only five percent of cases are directly inherited, prostate cancer that runs in families (familial prostate cancer) accounts for about 20 percent of cases.

A mutation in a gene located on chromosome 17 increases the risk of prostate cancer by 44 percent. Other genes that may cause an increased risk of heritable prostate cancer include HPC1, HPC2, HPCX, and CAPB.

A disorder similar to hereditary breast and ovarian cancer in women, **hereditary breast and ovarian cancer (HBOC) syndrome** also occurs in men, though posing breast and prostate cancer risk instead. A predisposition to this syndrome in both sexes is primarily due to mutations in the BRCA1 and BRCA2 genes.

Working with toxic materials — like cadmium, zinc, rubber, and oil refining processes — also has been linked to prostate cancer. Obesity and a high-fat diet may contribute to its development as well. Trichomoniasis, a common sexually transmitted disease (STD) increases prostate cancer risk as well as cancer-related mortality rate.

Outcome and Survival Rates

Almost 2.8 million men in the United States today are prostate cancer survivors. As with most cancers, the survival rate is dependent on how early the cancer is treated. More than 90 percent of all prostate cancers are discovered in the local or regional stage, for which the five-year survival rate is nearly 100 percent (Stages I–III). However, if the cancer spreads to distant organs (Stage IV), the five-year survival rate drops to 28 percent.

"Prostate cancer is not a death sentence. When prostate cancer is caught early, the outcome is superb, but you have to find a doctor who will fight for you," says Dr. David Samadi, who is chief of robotic surgery at Lenox Hill Hospital in New York City.

The PSA Test

One of the biggest controversies in prostate cancer is the use of the PSA blood test for screening. The PSA test measures the blood level of **prostate specific antigen**, a protein produced by the prostate gland. The higher a man's PSA level, or score, the more likely it is that he has prostate cancer.

Adult men usually have PSA levels below four nanograms per milliliter (ng/mL). A PSA level between four and 10 is borderline-high and suggests a 25 percent cancer risk. A PSA above 10 is high, and suggests a risk above 67 percent.

Other factors are taken into consideration as well. PSA levels rise naturally with age, which is known as **PSA velocity**. A higher-than-normal rise in this number increases the likelihood of prostate cancer. There is also an indicator known as **free PSA** that is taken into consideration. One form of PSA attaches to blood proteins and another circulates freely in the blood. Men with prostate cancer have lesser amounts of free PSA than men without prostate cancer.

For the past several years, the PSA test has been used as a screening tool to diagnose prostate cancer in healthy men, which has led to about one million men undergoing biopsies each year, but only one-fifth of them have resulted in a finding of cancer. This is because many other factors can lead to high a high PSA score, including a past infection of the prostate gland, interrupted blood flow to the gland, or benign enlargement (hyperplasia) of the prostate (BPH), which is common in men as they age.

Because of the great possibility of false findings, which can result in anxiety and unnecessary treatment, PSA screening is one of the hottest controversies in medicine. The US Preventive Services Task Force no longer recommends that healthy men be screened, and the American Urological Association (AUA) has scaled back its recommendation to endorse the test only for men aged 55 to 69, following a discussion of risks versus benefits with their doctor.

Dr. Robert C. Flanigan, professor of urology and chair of the department at Loyola University Medical Center, disagrees with the recommendation of the US Preventive Services Task Force. He contends that PSA screening does save lives: "No doubt there is a problem in that we have overtreated some prostate cancer cases, and there have been some side effects from treatment in cases where the disease is not life-threatening. But before screening became widespread, 25 to 30 percent of men undergoing surgery had cancer that had spread and was incurable. Now that rate has dropped to approximately two percent when PSA is routinely done," he says.

DID YOU KNOW . . .

While you may hear a lot about the controversy over the use of PSA testing, you should bear in mind that this issue pertains only to screening. If you have been diagnosed with prostate cancer, remember that the PSA test is an important tool that is used to gauge the effectiveness of treatment and also in determining if the cancer has returned.

Types of Prostate Cancer

Nearly all prostate cancer tumors — 95 percent — are adenocarcinomas, which is a malignant tumor that begins in the tissues of a gland. The remainder is comprised of different types of rare cancers.

Stages of Prostate Cancer

As with other forms of cancer, the stage at which prostate cancer is diagnosed predicates its prognosis and treatment. The staging of prostate cancer, however, is particularly complex because it is often very difficult to determine how risky a tumor could become. Therefore, there may be differences in prognosis based on other factors, including the volume or size of the tumor, the part of the prostate in which it is located, the PSA score, the number of cores (samples from a hollow needle biopsy) in which the prostate cancer is found, and the tumor grade.

Today, most physicians stage prostate cancers using the TNM system: **T (tumor)**, **N (node)**, and **M (metastasis)**. For patients with presumed localized prostate cancer, stages T1 through T4 indicate whether or not the cancer can be felt by the physician, and if so, the size and location of the tumor. The node categories NX, N0, and N1 indicate whether or not the cancer has spread to the lymph nodes. And finally, metastasis stages M0 or M1 are determined based on whether or not the cancer has spread past the lymph nodes, and if so, to which parts of the body/organs it has spread.

Grading Prostate Cancer: The Gleason Score

The Gleason score is a formula used to determine the aggressiveness of the prostate cancer. In the Gleason scoring system, two numbers are assigned to each biopsy containing a cancer. The first number is the grade (ranging from 1 through 5) of the tumor pattern making up the majority of the tumor, and the second number refers to any other tumor pattern that may be present. If the tumor appears to be uniform (containing only one pattern), the same number is simply repeated. For example, if there is only one tumor pattern in the sample and that tumor pattern is graded at 3, the Gleason score is 6: 3+3=6. The highest score (10) is reserved for the most varied cancer samples. The greater the variety of patterns found in a sample, the more aggressive the case.

Stage Grouping

When the cancer is staged using the TNM system, a Gleason score is applied, and a PSA level has been determined, this data is taken together to form more detailed sub-stages of the broader ones listed here:

STAGE I

Cancer is found in the prostate only, usually during another medical procedure. It cannot be felt during a digital rectal exam or seen on imaging tests. It also has a lower Gleason score, meaning the cells resemble healthy cells and the cancer is more likely to grow slowly.

STAGE II

The cancer is more advanced but has not spread beyond the prostate. This stage is divided into Stage IIA and Stage II B. There are several different classifications, depending on the PSA levels, Gleason scores, and the amount of tumors found on one lobe (of which there are four) of the prostate.

STAGE III

The cancer has spread beyond the prostate's outer layer and also may have spread to the seminal vesicles, the pair of tube-like glands located behind the bladder that secrete fluid into the ejaculatory tract. The PSA can be any level and the Gleason score can range from 2 to 10.

STAGE IV

Again, the PSA can be any level and the Gleason score can range from 2 to 10. In addition, the cancer may have spread beyond the seminal vesicles to nearby organs, such as the rectum, bladder, or pelvic wall, to nearby lymph nodes, or to distant parts of the body, which may include bones or additional lymph nodes.

Signs and Symptoms

In its early stages, prostate cancer usually does not cause symptoms. Later on, when symptoms do occur, they may include the following:

- Frequent urination, especially at night
- Trouble initiating or holding back urine flow
- Weak or interrupted urine flow
- Pain or burning during urination
- Blood in the urine
- Blood in the seminal fluid
- Pain the lower back, pelvis, or upper thighs

Specific Diagnostic Tests
DIGITAL RECTAL EXAM
The doctor inserts a lubricated, gloved finger into the rectum to check the prostate, feeling for bumps and other abnormalities.

IMAGING TESTS
Once a diagnosis of prostate cancer is confirmed, imaging tests, including **CT** (computed tomography) scan, **MRI** (magnetic resonance imaging), and **bone scans** are used to see if it has spread. (When prostate cancer spreads, it often targets the bones, hence the necessity for a bone scan.) A **transrectal ultrasound** may be performed — a procedure in which the doctor inserts a probe into the rectum that uses sound waves to provide an image of the prostate. In some cases, biopsies may be done with ultrasound direction after an MRI of the prostate is added into the ultrasound image.

BIOPSY
Tissue samples are required to confirm a diagnosis of prostate cancer. The core needle biopsy is the type generally used in prostate cancer. The doctor quickly inserts a thin, hollow needle through the wall of the rectum into the prostate gland. When the needle is pulled out it removes a small cylinder (core) of prostate tissue. This is repeated from eight to 18 times, but most urologists will take about 12 samples. This procedure is used to confirm a diagnosis of prostate cancer as well as stage it, as the number of core samples that turn up positive for cancer is an indication of the disease's progression.

Treatments
EARLY STAGE PROSTATE CANCER
The controversy over PSA screening is not the only debate when it comes to dealing with this disease. For most types of cancers, the treatment protocol is well-defined. But, when it comes to prostate cancer, even top experts can disagree on which type of treatment is the best for early stage, localized prostate cancer.

The following are the alternatives that will be offered to you based on the philosophy of your healthcare practitioner:

- Active surveillance (known also as "watchful waiting")

- Surgical, radical prostatectomy (open, robotic, or laparoscopic)
- Radiation (brachytherapy or external beam)

IS SURVEILLANCE OR TREATMENT BEST IN EARLY STAGE?

What makes dealing with early stage prostate cancer so difficult is that currently there is no foolproof way to determine whether it is an indolent (slow-growing) disease, or if/when it may suddenly turn aggressive and life-threatening.

"Most urologists classify prostate cancer as low-, intermediate-, and high-risk, but even among low-risk patients there are different factors, such as age, etc., that can be very important. Often there is no right or wrong decision as to the type of treatment, so a physician has to outline the positive and negatives with each approach, and every case requires a personal decision," notes Dr. Flanigan.

"When patients are newly diagnosed with prostate cancer, there is a lot of information coming at them fast and furiously. I discuss the options with my patients according to their individual case, and I also provide them with a written explanation of their options so that they have an opportunity to consider it and also talk it over their loved ones," he adds.

GOOD ADVICE

If you are diagnosed with early stage prostate cancer, don't panic and and risk making a hasty decision when it comes to treatment. Make sure that your doctor explains all your choices and provides you with written information. Then take some time to consider your options, do plenty of research, and discuss the alternatives with your spouse and/or loved ones.

ACTIVE SURVEILLANCE

Although this option is often termed **watchful waiting**, or **monitoring**, the term "active surveillance" is more accurate, because it does not mean just sitting back to see if the cancer becomes aggressive. Instead, if you opt for this choice, you would undergo a schedule of periodic PSA tests and digital rectal exams. You would also have undergone a biopsy to obtain as much information as possible about the tumor and how it may be changing over time.

Although active surveillance is a popular option, care must be taken in making certain that the appropriate patients are selected, and that the specifics of the particular patient are taken into account, including age, the size of the tumor and Gleason score, and also any co-existing medical conditions. Such a course might be preferable for a man who is of an advanced age, with another serious medical condition that may end up claiming his life instead, as opposed to a younger man with no co-existing conditions, who could possibly die of prostate cancer should his tumor become aggressive.

PROSTATECTOMY

The surgical removal of the prostate gland is generally the treatment of choice for prostate cancer patients who are younger, or also for those who are older but are in very good physical condition, with a normal remaining lifespan that would exceed at least 10 years.

This surgery, which is done with the goal of curing the cancer, is called a radical prostatectomy. It can be done in two ways: either **open**, which means using a traditional surgical procedure that involves a large incision, or performed **laparoscopically**, which utilizes a series of small incisions instead.

Robotic-Assisted Prostatectomy

Laparoscopic surgery to remove the prostate can be done by hand, like traditional surgery, but increasingly the doctors who perform it use a robotic system. Done this way, the doctor guides the robotic arms that wield the surgical tools.

Radical Open Prostatectomy

In open surgery, the surgeon makes a vertical eight-inch to 10-inch incision to reach the prostate gland. The incision may be made either in the lower belly between the navel and pelvic bone **(retropubic approach)**, or in the perineum, which is the area between the anus and the scrotum **(perineal approach)**. The lymph nodes are often also removed from this area so they can be tested for cancer; however, if the lymph nodes are believed to be free of cancer based on the grade of the cancer and results of the PSA test, the surgeon may opt not to remove lymph nodes.

Laparoscopic Prostatectomy

Similar to radical open prostatectomy, this type of surgery is performed to remove the prostate gland, along with all of the cancer.

The surgeon makes a series of small incisions, and then uses special instruments to reach in and remove the prostate.

Robotic-Assisted Laparoscopic Radical Prostatectomy

This technique, which is becoming increasingly popular, is performed through small incisions in the belly. The surgeon sits at a computer and, using hand and wrist movements, remotely operates robotic arms that translate his motions into finer and more precise action in order to remove the prostate and other cancerous tissue.

COMPLICATIONS OF RADICAL PROSTATECTOMY

Complications that occur during or early after prostatectomy most often include bleeding, infection, and pain. The major long-term complications associated with prostatectomy are loss of the ability to have erections and loss of bladder control (incontinence).

In general, a robotic prostatectomy causes less bleeding and less pain, but the control of the cancer, sexual, and urinary side effects can be similar to a radical (open) prostatectomy. The robotic procedure has not been available for as long as radical (open) prostatectomy, so there is less information on long-term results.

"Robotic surgery has been marketed extremely well. There aren't any large, randomized studies that compare robotic and open surgery, so when you look at the data, you can come to different conclusions," says Dr. Flanigan.

In selecting the type of procedure to opt for, it's very important to make sure that the surgeon is extremely experienced with the specific treatment technique.

"Unfortunately, there is also no central clearinghouse that offers data regarding a surgeon's experience level. So you should choose your prospective surgeon carefully. Ask the surgeon such questions as, 'What types of cases make up your practice?' and, 'How many of these procedures have you done or do you do each year?' It is generally important to choose a surgeon who performs these procedures on a regular basis. In many cases, if a surgeon does only a relatively small number of the procedure you need, his or her skills may not be at the highest level," Dr. Flanigan says.

Radiation

Radiation therapy is the use of high-energy rays to kill cancer cells. Radiation can be used to treat early-stage prostate cancer as part of the first-line therapy (along with hormone therapy) for cancers not completely removed by surgery, and for recurrent prostate cancer.

BRACHYTHERAPY

Brachytherapy is the insertion of radioactive sources, called seeds, directly into the prostate gland, supplying a high dose of radiation to the cancer itself without disturbing nearby, unaffected tissues.

EXTERNAL-BEAM RADIATION THERAPY

This is the most common type of radiation performed to treat prostate cancer. External-beam radiation therapy focuses a beam of radiation on the area with the cancer.

Intensity-Modulated Radiation Therapy (IMRT)

This type of external-beam radiation therapy involves CT scans to form a three-dimensional picture of the prostate cancer before treatment, which is used to determine how much radiation is needed to destroy it. This way, high doses of radiation can be directed at the prostate without increasing the risk of damaging nearby organs.

Proton Therapy

Also called proton-beam radiation therapy, this type of external-beam radiation therapy destroys cancer cells with the use of protons (positively charged particles) rather than X-ray radiation, which can be more harmful to nearby organs.

HORMONE THERAPY

This mode of therapy relies on the removal or suppression of the male hormone, testosterone, which fuels the growth of prostate cancer. This can be accomplished either by removing the testicles (orchiectomy), or by injecting **Lupron**, a substance that suppresses testosterone. This treatment is generally used either prior to surgical removal of the prostate or to treat symptoms when the cancer is advanced.

CRYOTHERAPY

This type of treatment involves the use of freezing techniques to destroy the prostate. This is not a treatment for primary prostate cancer, but it is an option for treating recurrent prostate cancer, especially if radiation does not kill enough cancer cells.

CHEMOTHERAPY

Sometimes chemotherapy is used for prostate cancer, but not as much as it is used to treat other types of cancer.

IMMUNOTHERAPY

Researchers have long hoped to discover a cancer "vaccine" that would stimulate the immune system and, finally in 2010, the FDA approved the first one: sipuleucel (Provenge). This treatment is for men with prostate cancer that has spread but has not responded to hormone therapy and is causing few symptoms. Other types of immunological treatments for prostate cancer are currently in the testing stages.

Brain Cancer

10

NOT SO VERY LONG ago, brain cancer was considered incurable. But, although brain cancer remains one of the most serious forms of cancer, the survival outlook is brighter now than ever before, as voice coach Brett Johnson learned. In 2009, not only was he diagnosed with a brain tumor, but it was a particularly aggressive type. "I kind of fell apart," he recalls. But Johnson quickly rallied and today, after two surgeries and chemotherapy, he is back at his studio working with his students. "Most people with my brain tumor don't live more than 10 or 12 years, but considering that the prognosis used to be measured in months, I keep thinking, 'This isn't what is going to kill me,' and I feel very certain that is true," he says.

What Is Brain Cancer?

The term "brain cancer" can be confusing, because it's sometimes used to refer to cancer that develops in the brain (known also as a "primary" brain tumor) and also for cancer that has spread to the brain (metastatic brain tumor), which tends to occur most often in lung and breast cancer. Depending on the location of the cancer, as tumors grow they crowd brain tissue, interfering with key brain functions, such as memory, muscle movements, sight, speech, sensation, and other bodily systems and functions.

Statistics

Although it is difficult to determine the number of adult brain cancer survivors because the data is usually mixed with that of children, it's been estimated that there are about 690,000 people in the United States living with brain cancer.

Although brain tumors can occur at any age, adult brain tumors commonly occur in people between 50 and 60 years old. About 23,500 people are diagnosed with a brain tumor each year, and roughly 14,500 will unfortunately succumb to the disease. Approximately half of all brain cancers are nonmalignant, meaning abnormal cells are noncancerous and incapable of spreading, but they can still be life-threatening. Most types of primary brain tumors occur in men, with the exception of meningiomas, which are more common to women.

Outcome and Survival Rates

Decades ago, brain cancer was considered incurable, with virtually all patients expected to survive only a matter of months, not years. But that picture has changed, and many brain cancer patients are living longer and with a significantly better quality of life than in the past.

"It's important to realize that brain cancer isn't the death sentence it once was. There is hope," says Lee M. Tessler, MD, a neurosurgeon and executive director of the Long Island Brain Tumor Center.

For most types of cancer, the prognosis depends on the stage in which the cancer is diagnosed, but this is not the case with brain tumors because they stay contained within the skull and do not spread to other organs. But such tumors can grow in size and endanger other brain functions, affecting senses, bodily systems, and organs. "Since brain cancer doesn't spread to other parts of the body, we don't talk about stages, we talk about it in terms of grades or aggressiveness. Knowing the grade of a brain tumor is all we need to do to stop its growth," says Dr. Tessler.

The survival rate for people with brain tumors depends on many factors, including the type of tumor, its size and location (which affects whether it can be surgically removed), and its grade, as well as the age and medical condition of the patient.

Brain cancer survival rates vary widely, depending on its type. Meningiomas are tumors that originate from the meninges, which are the three protective layers that cover the brain and the spinal cord. The vast majority of meningiomas (some 90 percent), which are considered Grade I, are cured through surgical removal, with no recurrence seen in 93 percent of patients after 10 years. On the other end of the spectrum are the gliomas, which are faster growing and tend to be more diffuse, or spread out over the brain. The outlook for patients with gliomas is generally poorer, but even progress in this type of cancer has been made in terms of quality of life.

Types of Brain Cancer

There are many, many different types and subtypes of primary brain cancer, but the common types fall into the two major groups previously described: meningiomas and gliomas. Pituitary and nerve sheath tumors make up the remainder of cases.

MENINGIOMAS

This is the most common adult form of brain cancer, and accounts for 34 percent of all primary brain tumors. This slow-growing cancer originating in the meninges is not malignant, but masses can grow large enough to be life-threatening and must be treated. Most low-grade meningiomas that are located in easy-to-reach areas can be treated successfully with surgery and radiation, but higher grade, more aggressive tumors are difficult to eradicate and are more life-threatening.

GLIOMA

This is the general term that refers to tumors that start in the **glial cells**, which are the gluey, spongy cells that protect and support the brain's neurons, providing them with stability, insulating each from the other, delivering them oxygen and nutrients, destroying toxins, and removing dead neurons. The glial cells can give rise to a variety of tumors, ranging from benign to malignant. Types of gliomas include: **glioblastomas, astrocytomas,**

oligodendrogliomas, and **ependymomas**. Gliomas make up 30 percent of all brain and central nervous system tumors, and 80 percent of all malignant brain tumors.

MIXED GLIOMAS

These are tumors in which two different types of tumor cells — oligodendrocytes and astrocytes — are involved. This mixed tumor is referred to as an oligoastrocytoma. The Grade II level of this tumor is very slow-growing, and a cure is sometimes achieved. The Grade III level, called **anaplastic oligoastrocytoma,** is very aggressive and prone to spreading, making the prognosis unfavorable.

PITUITARY GLAND CANCER

Known as the "master" endocrine gland, this pea-sized gland, located behind the eyes and at the base of the front of the brain, produces hormones that govern many of the body's functions, like growth, blood pressure, sexual function, and thyroid activity, just to name several. Most pituitary gland tumors are benign, and the condition is actually quite rare, accounting for about 10 percent of all primary brain cancers. Women of childbearing age are more likely to develop pituitary gland cancer.

NERVE SHEATH CANCER

Nerve sheath (coating around nerve fibers) cancer accounts for about nine percent of brain cancer cases. This form of cancer arises in the nerve cells of the peripheral nervous system, which connects the brain and spinal cord with rest of the body, such as the limbs.

Grades of Brain Cancer

Because brain cancer does not spread outside of the brain, it is categorized according to "grade" instead of "stage." The grade of the brain tumor denotes how fast-growing it is and how dangerous it is likely to become.

GRADE I

The tissue is benign. The cells look nearly like normal brain cells, and they grow slowly. Generally, Grade I tumors have the most favorable outcome, although much depends on where the tumor is located. A Grade I brain tumor may still require aggressive treatment if it is located in an important area of the brain where minimal growth (if at all) would cause problems.

GRADE II

The tissue is malignant. The cells look less like normal cells than do the cells in a Grade I tumor.

GRADE III

These are cells that look very different from normal cells. The abnormal cells are actively growing.

GRADE IV

The malignant tissue has cells that look most abnormal and tend to grow quickly.

Signs and Symptoms

- Headaches that are often severe upon awakening or that worsen with activity, but lessen as the day wears on

- Seizures, also called convulsions, are sudden involuntary movements of person's muscles. There are many different types of seizures, with symptoms ranging from muscle twitches to loss of consciousness and control of bodily movements. Seizures can also cause changes in smell, vision, or hearing (without losing consciousness), or the stoppage of breathing for short periods of time

- Vomiting, usually after awakening, with or without nausea

- Weakness or loss of feeling in the arms or legs

- Difficulty walking or clumsiness

- One-sided muscle weakness

- Difficulty speaking or swallowing

- Ringing or buzzing in the ears

- Vision changes

- Changes in personality or memory change

- Drowsiness or fatigue

Specific Diagnostic Tests

This is a rundown on tests that are specifically performed to diagnose brain cancer. For more information on general testing for cancer, see chapter 2.

NEUROLOGICAL EXAMINATION

Diagnosing a brain tumor usually begins when a patient starts to experience symptoms and goes to the family doctor or internist, who performs a neurological examination. These are basic checks of the eyes, hearing, reflexes, balance and coordination, sense of touch and smell, as well as tests to check movement of facial muscles, tongue and gag reflex, and the head. Simple tests to check for thinking problems, memory, and abstract thinking may also be performed. If any abnormalities are found, the patient is referred to a neurologist for further testing.

BRAIN SCAN

A brain scan involves the taking of multiple digital images to compile a picture of the internal anatomy of the brain. Sometimes, a contrast dye is injected into a vein and flows into the brain tissue, which highlights any abnormalities.

IMAGING TESTS

Computed tomography (CT or CAT) scans, magnetic resonance imaging (MRI), and other non-invasive imaging tests provide images of the brain that can be used in treatment.

A **cerebral arteriogram**, also known as a **cerebral angiogram**, is an X-ray or series of X-rays of the head that shows the arteries in the brain. A **myelogram** is a test in which a dye is injected into the fluid surrounding the spinal cord, which then provides an outline of it on an X-ray. These days, lumbar punctures are more commonly performed instead.

LUMBAR PUNCTURE

More frequently referred to as a **spinal tap**, this is a procedure in which a needle is used to take a sample of the **cerebral spinal fluid (CSF)** to look for tumor cells, blood, or tumor markers.

BIOPSY

A biopsy is the final diagnostic test, which involves the extraction of a sample of the cells from the tumor and the examination under a microscope. This is the most accurate way to confirm the diagnosis of a brain tumor and also determine its grade.

BLOOD TESTS AND TUMOR MARKERS

Brain tumors can secrete substances that can be used to identify specific genes, proteins, and other factors, such as tumor markers, which are unique to the mass. Such tumor markers may be found in the blood, urine, CSF, and other types of bodily fluids. The results can be used to customize a treatment unique to the tumor.

Treatments

SURGERY

Surgery is the oldest and most common form of treatment for brain cancer. The goal of brain surgery is to remove the entire tumor, if possible. Even if that proves impossible, the partial removal of the tumor can make treatment easier and more effective.

Fortunately, over the years, much progress has been made, so tumors can be removed far more carefully. "In terms of surgery, we used to be happy when someone survived, but they ended up looking like stroke victims. Now we have really good, high-tech ways of getting to the tumor, taking it out, and sparing the brain tissue around it," Dr. Tessler says.

Another key improvement is **intraoperative brain mapping**. This is an innovative computer technique that enables surgeons to see a map of the patient's individual brain, which shows exactly where are the vital areas are, including vision, hearing, taste,

GOOD ADVICE

If you are diagnosed with brain cancer, don't panic. Unless it's an emergency, you have time to research and select the best place to get treated. Brain cancer in adults is rare, and some forms are much rarer than others, so make sure the team you select is experienced in treating that form of cancer. This doesn't necessarily mean you must utilize a major cancer treatment center, but it does mean that the doctors must be skilled in treating the type of brain cancer you have.

touch, movement, and language centers. "With the brain, you can't do the exploratory procedures you would do in other parts of the body because you would damage brain tissue. So we now have this technique that creates a three-dimensional picture of the brain, showing the tumor, so when I'm in the operating room, I can look at the picture on a computer screen and know exactly what I need to do," says Dr. Tessler.

In addition, there are also now ways to perform brain surgery while the patient is kept awake and able to respond. "Unlike the rest of the body, the brain does not have pain receptors, so the surgery is actually pain-free. Because of this, I can ask the patient to speak or move, and so I can see those vital areas during the surgery and avoid them," Dr. Tessler adds.

As a patient, Johnson concurs. Although he found the idea of brain surgery very worrisome, he was surprised it was not more painful. "There are less nerves in your head than in other parts of your body, so even though my head hurt, I think that when you have surgery elsewhere in your body, the pain is probably more severe."

STEREOTACTIC RADIATION

Stereotactic radiation, or **stereotaxy**, is a way to eradicate a tumor using radiation. The procedure goes by different names, such as **Gamma Knife**, **Novalis**, and **Cyberknife**, depending on the device manufacturer. Basically, though, this procedure combines sophisticated computerized software to target radiation to the brain and eradicate the tumor while sparing the delicate surrounding brain tissue. This method is used on less aggressive brain tumors, as well as cancer that has metastasized, or spread, to the brain from other sites, like lung or breast cancer.

CHEMOTHERAPY

Chemotherapy is sometimes used to treat brain cancer, but does not play as much of a role in treatment as it does in other forms of cancer because the drugs cannot pass the blood-brain barrier, which is the network of tightly packed cells that prevent foreign substances in the bloodstream from entering the brain. Also, not all types of brain tumors respond to chemotherapy. So, for these reasons, surgery and radiation are the primary ways of treating brain cancer. However, the anti-cancer drug **temozolomide** (**Temodar**, **Temodal**, and **Temcad**) is used in the treatment of some brain cancers, especially along with radiation, because studies have shown it may improve survival and quality of life.

Other Drugs

Additional types of drugs used to fight brain cancer include: **bevacizumab (Avastin)**, which blocks the growth of blood vessels that feed the tumor; **everolimus (Afinitor)**, which is a targeted therapy; and possibly **imatinib mesylate (Gleevec)**, the leukemia drug that researchers are currently testing as a treatment for brain cancer.

Immunotherapy

Immunotherapy is the use of substances to stimulate the body's immune response and marshal it to stop the growth or spread of cancer. Immunotherapy is one of the frontiers in treating brain cancer, and is being looked upon as a promising future treatment, but it is also being used now. One of the newest immunologic agents for brain cancer and the first of its kind is **pembrolizumab (Keytruda)**, approved by the FDA in 2014.

> **GOOD ADVICE**
>
> Don't let brain cancer rob you of your quality of life. Measures like physical activity can make a big difference, both in terms of survival and quality of life, so make sure that the treatment center you choose has a physical therapy program for brain cancer patients.

Cancer That Spreads to the Brain

This chapter is focused on cancer that begins in the brain, but a question that continually arises is what to do about cancer that spreads to the brain, from the lung or in the case of melanoma, for instance.

Whole brain radiation used to be a standard treatment for such metastasis, but many studies have found that this treatment causes devastating effects in terms of the patient's thinking and functioning abilities without prolonging life, so the stereotactic techniques previously described are now being found preferable.

11

Bladder Cancer

DESPITE REPEATED ROUNDS OF antibiotics, Anna
Strazzante's urinary tract infections kept coming back. "Some
women just get UTIs," her doctor told her. But Anna wasn't satisfied. As a physical therapist, she did have knowledge of medicine,
so finally she asked her doctor if he thought she might have cancer, but he brushed her off. When she started urinating blood, she
called her doctor's office again, but the nurse was unconcerned.
Finally, Anna insisted on testing, and bladder cancer was the diagnosis. Now, five years later, Anna is cancer-free. But she tells
everyone she knows, "Listen to your intuition. If it seems to you
that something is wrong, question it!"

What Is Bladder Cancer?

The bladder is an expandable, balloon-shaped organ that stores
the urine that the kidneys excrete through tubes (one for each
kidney) called ureters. Bladder cancer develops when the normal

cells of the bladder's four-layered lining begin to grow uncontrollably and form a tumor. Like other tumors, a bladder tumor can be benign, or become malignant, and spread from the bladder to other organs as well.

Statistics

There are roughly 73,000 new cases of bladder cancer diagnosed in the United States each year. The disease occurs far more often in men, who will develop an estimated 55,000 cases, compared to 18,000 in women; this translates to one in 26 men versus one in 90 women. Caucasians are diagnosed with bladder cancer almost twice as often as African-Americans, but the latter are slightly more likely to have their cancers diagnosed at a more advanced stage. Asians have the lowest rate of bladder cancer. Overall, about nine out of 10 people with bladder cancer are over the age of 55, with the average person being diagnosed at age 73.

People develop bladder cancer even if they have no predisposition to the disease, but there are several risk factors that increase the probability. Some genetic disorders can increase risk, including **Lynch syndrome**, or HNPCC (see chapter 8), which is primarily associated with an increased colon and endometrial cancer risk. Inheriting certain rare, specific birth defects can also increase the chances of developing bladder cancer.

Occupational exposure to carcinogens, or cancer-causing chemicals, also ups bladder cancer risk. This danger especially pertains to painters, machinists, printers, hairdressers (due to heavy exposure to hair dyes), and truck drivers, most likely because of exposure to diesel fumes.

But genetic syndromes, birth defects, or occupational chemical exposure are not the major cause of bladder cancer; smoking is. "When it comes to smoking, bladder cancer is very similar to lung cancer," says Blaine Kristo, MD, a urologist who specializes in bladder cancer at Mercy Medical Center in Baltimore, Maryland.

Smokers are three times more likely to develop bladder cancer, and smoking is responsible for half of the bladder cancers in both men and women. This is because when you smoke, you inhale cancer-causing chemicals into your lungs, which then get into your blood and travel to the kidneys. The kidneys filter out these chemicals, and they end up concentrated in the urine, where they sit in the bladder, damaging the lining of the organ and leading to cancerous changes.

"In fact, smoking is so closely linked to bladder cancer that, even when people are diagnosed with it, they find it tough to give up the habit," says Dr. Kristo. "Many patients are still smoking when they come to see me. I tell them they have to do everything they can to stop; this is important. In the case of many types of cancer, like lung cancer, once a patient is diagnosed and stops smoking, it may be too late. But this is not true of bladder cancer. Since most bladder cancer is superficial when it's diagnosed, a cure is very likely."

DID YOU KNOW . . .

The risk of superficial (or early stage) bladder cancer recurrence is very high, but quitting smoking reduces this risk. "There aren't many cancers in which quitting smoking directly affects the outcome, but it does in bladder cancer. If you have noninvasive bladder cancer and you quit, you can reduce the risk of recurrence by about 30 percent," Dr. Kristo says.

Outcome and Survival Rates

More than 500,000 people in the United States today are bladder cancer survivors. As with most cancers, the survival rate is dependent on how early the cancer is treated, ranging from 98 percent in those whose cancers are caught the earliest, to 63 percent for Stage II. The survival rate for Stage III bladder cancer is 46 percent, and for Stage IV is 15 percent if the bladder cancer has spread to distant organs. Again, it is important to remember that there are people today surviving bladder cancer no matter what stage their cancer was diagnosed.

Types of Bladder Cancer

Bladder cancer is divided in types according to how the cells appear. The vast majority of bladder cases are known as "transitional cell bladder cancer," comprising 95 percent of all cases. The remaining five percent include squamous cell carcinoma, adenocarcinoma, small cell carcinoma, and sarcomas. (Sarcomas are treated differently and discussed in detail in chapter 16.)

TRANSITIONAL CELL BLADDER CANCER

The most common of all bladder cancers in the United States, transitional cell cancer arises in the **urothelium**, or **transitional**

epithelium, which is the bladder wall's innermost lining. These cells can also be present in the linings of the ureters and urethra. Transitional cells are very elastic in nature — they stretch as the bladder expands, and shrink when it's empty; the transitional cell is also capable of changing shape. Although the transitional is the only type of cell involved in this major form of bladder cancer, it can take on various forms. Transitional cell carcinoma of the bladder is also subdivided into two types:

- **Papillary bladder cancer** starts in the urothelium, but grows into the bladder cavity, remaining attached by a mushroom-like stalk. Since this type of cancer grows in toward the hollow center of the bladder, it is noninvasive to the other layers of the bladder. Papillary carcinoma has a very low malignancy rate and is easily operable. Quite often, tumors never return.

- **Nonpapillary bladder cancer** is composed of flat lesions. When they occur on the urothelium, they are considered noninvasive; however, they can become invasive, or spread to the outer layers of the bladder. Nonpapillary carcinomas are also referred to as "flat carcinoma in situ."

SUPERFICIAL BLADDER CANCER

This type makes up 75 percent of all transitional bladder cancer cases. This is a common form of bladder cancer that occurs in the lining of the bladder. Although it does not spread, it can recur after treatment.

INVASIVE BLADDER CANCER

This is the most dangerous form of the disease. It can grow into the lining of the bladder and burrow into the muscle wall.

Stages of Bladder Cancer
STAGE 0

In this earliest stage, cancerous cells are found only in the surface of the bladder's lining. The survival rate for this earlier stage of cancer is 98 percent. This is also known as cancer in situ, or non-invasive bladder cancer.

STAGE I

Cancerous cells are found in the thin lining of the bladder, but they have not spread to the muscle of the bladder.

STAGE II

The cancer has spread to the muscle of the bladder. Most bladder cancers are diagnosed at this stage because it is when blood is most likely to show up in the urine.

STAGE III

The cancer has spread through the muscular wall to the tissue that surrounds the bladder. In men, this would be the prostate gland, and in women, the uterus or vagina.

STAGE IV

The cancer has spread to the abdominal wall or the pelvis, and possibly to nearby lymph nodes and distant organs.

Signs and Symptoms

- Blood in the urine is the main clinical sign of bladder cancer. "The problem is denial. Many people see blood in their urine and they know that it could mean something bad so they don't show up until several months later and by that time the cancer has spread to the muscle. So the key is getting checked out promptly. This is especially important in older people with a history of smoking, even if that habit took place 20 years ago," Dr. Kristo notes.

- Feeling irritation, discomfort, or pain urinating

- Needing to urinate more frequently than usual

- Feeling the need to empty your bladder without results

- Needing to strain (bear down) when urinating

- Lower back pain

- A recurrent or treatment-resistant UTI is being recognized as a potential sign of bladder cancer. Though this cancer is more prevalent in men, women need to be especially vigilant in getting screened as chronic UTIs in females are often blamed on common causes (e. g., failure to urinate after sex, etc.).

Specific Diagnostic Tests

The following tests are specifically performed to diagnose bladder cancer. For more information on general testing for cancer, see chapter 2.

URINE CULTURE

The urine is checked to see if a bladder infection is responsible for symptoms.

CYTOSCOPY

An instrument called a cytoscope is inserted through the urethra to observe the inside surface of the bladder and collect samples of tissues that can be examined, or biopsied, to check for cancer. This is the most common bladder cancer test done. If abnormal tissue is found, a biopsy, called a **transurethral resection of bladder tumor (TURBT)**, is performed and the specimen is examined for cancer cells.

URINE TUMOR MARKER TESTS

This test checks the urine for specific substances (markers) that bladder tumors release. Although only a few bladder cancer tumor markers are currently known, this is a hot research area.

GOOD ADVICE

According to a UCLA study, almost half of bladder biopsies are of such low quality that the cancer may be inadequately treated, leading to a higher mortality rate. Therefore, if cancer is suspected, right from the start, it is crucial to see a urologist or urologic oncologist who is experienced in bladder cancer treatment.

IMAGING TESTS

Computed tomography (CT or CAT) scans and magnetic resonance imaging (MRI) are used to see if the cancer has spread. The most common imaging test, a CT urogram utilizes injected dye, then a CT scan to provide images of the urinary tract. Another test, the **retrograde pyelogram**, is used for those who have an allergy to X-ray dye.

Treatments

All cancer treatment depends on the stage at which it is diagnosed. "This is particularly important in bladder cancer because, although only one type of cell is involved, it can act as two different diseases, depending on its stage," says Dr. Kristo. "Stage 0 or I, remains on the surface of the bladder and can be removed. Once bladder cancer invades the muscle, however, both surgery to retain part or all of the bladder, along with chemotherapy and/or radiation, is needed."

If the cancer is on the superficial level, the urologist can treat it. But once it spreads to the muscular wall of the bladder, you need to see a urological oncologist who specializes in treating bladder cancer, or a urologist with a great deal of expertise in the disease. "A lot of urologists and urologic oncologists specialize in prostate cancer, so you need to find an expert at a hospital where a lot of bladder cancers are treated. The outcomes are better at a hospital that treats 100 cases a year versus just three," says Dr. Kristo.

Surgical Treatments

Bladder cancer is always treated with some form of surgery although the extent depends on the stage of the cancer.

TRANSURETHRAL SURGERY

Transurethral surgery is the most common form of treatment for bladder cancer and is the only treatment required for superficial bladder cancer, which is unlikely to spread. For this procedure, a wire-tipped tube called a **resectoscope** is passed into the bladder through the urethra, so no abdominal incision is needed. Cancerous cells are removed, and a laser is used to burn away any other suspicious tissue. This procedure can also be used to confirm a bladder cancer diagnosis as well as to stage the cancer.

CYSTECTOMY

This is the surgical procedure used for bladder cancers that are larger and have invaded the bladder wall. There are three types of cystectomies:

Partial Cystectomy

This surgery involves the removal of part of the bladder. It is a good choice if the cancer has entered the bladder wall, but is still small and confined to a single area. In this procedure, the tumor is removed, along with part of the bladder wall. The hole in the bladder wall is then closed. This procedure is appropriate only for small cancers that are not far advanced.

Simple Cystectomy

This procedure is used to remove the entire bladder.

Radical Cystectomy

This procedure involves the removal of the entire bladder, along with nearby lymph nodes, part of the urethra and any nearby organs that may contain cancer cells. In men, this would be the prostate, the seminal vesicles, and part of the vas deferens (the main duct through which the sperm travels). In women, the cervix, the uterus, the ovaries, the fallopian tubes, and part of the vagina are removed.

GOOD ADVICE

If you are scheduled for surgery, talk to your doctor about whether chemotherapy beforehand will help your outcome. —Dr. Kristo

BLADDER RECONSTRUCTION

When the bladder is removed, another way to store and remove urine from the body is needed. This requires reconstructive surgery, and many types are available. One option calls for the removal of short piece of the intestine, which is connected to the ureters, and then to the outside of the body. This option requires the use of a stoma (surgical opening). A small bag is connected to the stoma, which is emptied when it is full.

An alternative procedure is called a **continent diversion**. For this, a valve is created from a piece of intestine, which allows for urine to be stored in an internal pouch. It is drained several times each day by using a catheter.

There is also a newer method, called a **neobladder**, in which a sort of artificial bladder is created in the form of a urinary reservoir made of a piece of intestine. This option allows for normal urination. But although this may sound preferable, sometimes complications can occur, so it sometimes is better to go with the use of a stoma.

One of the key reasons why early stage superficial bladder cancer and later stage bladder cancer are treated so differently centers on the issue of removal of the bladder. In early stage bladder cancer, the superficial cancer can be removed and the bladder left in place. But when all or part of the bladder is removed, sometimes along with other organs like a man's prostate or a woman's reproductive organs, this can result in major problems like incontinence or sexual dysfunction.

"This is a big surgery, and it's a life-changing one, so it's critically important for patients to be plugged into a center that can provide not only excellent care, but also support for caregivers and patient support groups as well," says Dr. Kristo.

IMMUNOTHERAPY

This type of biological therapy uses the body's own immune system to fight cancer. Bladder cancer patients who undergo transurethral resection for superficial bladder cancer may be candidates for a biological treatment called **bacillus Calmette-Guérin (BCG)**, which helps prevent the cancer from recurring. For this, a live, weakened bacterial organism, BCG, is inserted into the bladder via catheter. The bacteria causes inflammation, stimulating the immune system to attack it and kill any remaining cancer cells.

> **GOOD ADVICE**
>
> If you've been diagnosed with invasive (likely to spread) bladder cancer, seek out a cancer treatment center or hospital with a specific invasive bladder cancer program. This can give you an edge not only during treatment, but also with regard to bladder reconstruction, which can be very important for your quality of life afterwards. A top or large cancer center is more likely to have such a program.

CHEMOTHERAPY

Chemotherapy is often used either before or after surgery. And like BCG, it is often used following transurethral surgery to wipe out any remaining microscopic cancer cells, but it can also be used beforehand, even in cases of advanced bladder cancer, to improve results after surgery.

"Previously, doctors have been reluctant to use chemotherapy in such cases, fearing the patient might be weakened too much and less able to withstand surgery, but research shows that this is a powerful strategy that can improve or extend survival, so it should be discussed," notes Dr. Kristo.

RADIATION

This common treatment uses high-energy radiation to kill cancer cells. It can be used as part of the treatment for early stage bladder cancer, as the main treatment for people with advanced bladder cancer who for various reasons aren't candidates for surgery, or to help prevent or treat symptoms caused by advanced bladder surgery. It can also be used to enhance the effects of chemotherapy.

12

Leukemia

JOANNE FILINA HADN'T FELT right in years, but her doctor had been brushing off her concerns. "Because I work in the medical field, he implied I was a hypochondriac," says Filina, who is an ultrasound technician. Finally, he referred her to a doctor who specializes in diseases of the blood and the diagnosis came back showing Joanne had an advanced form of leukemia.

"I remember my doctor saying words like 'no cure,' and 'this cancer doesn't respond to treatment.'" After local doctors told her she had only 18 months to live, she decided she had better be seen at a major cancer center. "There, they hit me hard with chemotherapy," she says. Now, nearly two years later, her leukemia is in remission.

What Is Leukemia?

All of our blood cells begin as stem cells, generated mainly in our bone marrow. As different genetically coded pathways lead each cell to maturity, some become white blood cells (meant to fight infection), some red blood cells (which carry oxygen), and others become platelets (responsible for clotting).

In the case of leukemia, our bone marrow produces abnormal white blood cells. These don't tend to die off like normal cells, and eventually crowd out healthy blood cells, preventing them from performing their essential life functions. Leukemia cells don't have the ability to fight infection like normal white cells, thus they compromise the entire body's immune system, collecting in the lymph nodes, spleen, and liver.

Though medical science is unsure of the exact trigger that causes the onset of the different types of leukemia, one thing is certain: environmental and genetic factors (chemical exposure or genetic abnormalities) seem to be the culprit. The word leukemia comes from the Greek *leukós* and *haîma*, which literally means "white blood."

Statistics

An estimated 45,000 new cases of adult leukemia cancer are diagnosed each year; almost 90 percent of cases occur in those over the age of 20, with the majority of sufferers aged 60 or older.

Men are about one-third more likely to develop leukemia than are women, and they are also more likely to die from it. Caucasians are more apt to get leukemia, with those of Jewish ancestry particularly susceptible to the disease.

People may develop leukemia even with no risk factors for the disease, but there are several factors that increase the probability. Some genetic syndromes can increase risk, such as Down syndrome, T-lymphotropic virus (HTLV-1), and HIV. Those who have undergone certain medical treatments are also at risk for developing leukemia because of repeated doses of radiation, especially certain cancer survivors who've received specific types of chemotherapy. As well, those who've suffered high-dose radiation exposure for any reason face a higher risk for the disease. Long-term or high-dose chemical exposure to benzene and other products containing this substance are also known to cause leukemia.

DID YOU KNOW . . .

Most people think of leukemia as a children's disease, but children account for less than 10 percent of leukemia diagnoses.

Outcome and Survival Rates

It is estimated that there are about 300,000 leukemia survivors in the United States. Treating leukemia is made especially complicated by the fact that there are many different forms of the disease, so deriving a prognosis from its various stages is markedly problematic. Generally, though, the outlook is fairly optimistic for leukemia patients because treatment has made remarkable progress over the past 50 years. In the early 1960s, the overall five-year survival rate was four percent. Today it stands at 64 percent.

Types of Leukemia

Leukemia is classified according to the type of white blood cell that is multiplying:

- Lymphocytes (immune system cells)
- Granulocytes (bacteria-destroying cells)
- Monocytes (macrophage-forming cells)

If the abnormal white blood cells are primarily granulocytes or monocytes, the leukemia is categorized as myelogenous, or **myeloid leukemia**. If the abnormal blood cells arise from bone marrow lymphocytes, the cancer is called **lymphocytic leukemia**.

There are four types of leukemia, which are divided into two broader categories: **acute leukemia** and **chronic leukemia.** The difference between the two is that the abnormal cells in acute leukemia appear more as stem cells, or blast cells, while in chronic leukemia, the abnormal cells appear to be closer in likeness to a normal white blood cell.

> **GOOD ADVICE**
>
> Because leukemia patients are likely to live many years after their treatment, they should also be seen at a center oriented specifically to their type of cancer; there, they are more likely to have programs for leukemia survivors. "People who are treated for leukemia may have major issues that may not manifest until years later so they need to be monitored, they need to be sure they get screening tests, and get the information and encouragement they need to live a healthy lifestyle," says Dr. Patrick Stiff, who is a hematological oncologist and director of Loyola University's Cardinal Bernardin Cancer Center.

ACUTE LEUKEMIA

Acute leukemia is a disease in which the bone marrow cells cannot mature properly so immature cells reproduce and build up in the bloodstream. Symptoms appear to come on suddenly, so patients feel ill right away. Types of acute leukemia include acute myeloid leukemia (AML) and acute lymphocytic leukemia (ALL). Acute leukemia means that the form of the disease is very dangerous and could be fatal within a few months if untreated; it must be treated immediately and intensively, eliminating all traces of the abnormal cells so the patient can be brought into remission.

Acute Myeloid Leukemia (AML)

AML is the most common form of adult leukemia. Most of those diagnosed are older (the average age of diagnosis is 65), and more men are affected than women. Generally, treatment can keep approximately 60 to 70 percent of people in remission, with an overall cure rate of 40 to 50 percent.

In a healthy individual, the bone marrow's myeloblast cells (or simply blast cells) mature into granulocytes, one of three major types of white blood cells, along with monocytes and lymphocytes. The main function of the granulocyte is to destroy bacteria. In the case of AML, blasts overproduce and do not grow into fully matured granulocytes; instead, these blasts become too numerous in the blood and bone marrow, crowding out healthy red and white blood cells, and platelets. As the blast cells build up, they hamper the body's ability to fight infection and prevent bleeding. Therefore, AML can become life-threatening if not treated quickly.

AML is also known as acute myelogenous leukemia, acute myelocytic leukemia, or acute nonlymphocytic leukemia.

Acute Lymphocytic Leukemia (ALL)

ALL is a situation in which the bone marrow manufactures too many lymphoblasts — lymphoid stem cells that evolve into blasts, but never fully mature into lymphocytes. As with AML, these immature cells crowd the marrow and blood, causing the disease to progress quickly and require prompt treatment. Lymphoblasts (abnormal lymph cells) may also collect in the lymphatic system and cause swelling of the lymph nodes. Some cells may invade other organs, including the brain, liver, spleen, or testicles in men. But unlike other types of cancer, the fact that ALL is found in other parts of the body does not mean that the cancer is in an advanced stage — acute leukemia is usually found throughout the body when it is diagnosed.

Caucasian males are most at risk for ALL, especially those over 70, those having undergone chemotherapy or radiation in the past, or individuals with Down syndrome or other genetic disorders.

CHRONIC LEUKEMIA

Chronic leukemia cells do not look as abnormal as those of acute leukemia; they can mature partially, but not completely. But even though the cells look fairly normal, they do not fight infection as well as normal white blood cells. The cells also live longer or don't die at all as healthy cells do, so they can crowd out normal cells. Chronic leukemia can develop slowly — sometimes over the course of years — and people may remain asymptomatic for a very long time. The two types of chronic leukemia are chronic lymphocytic leukemia (CML) and chronic myeloid leukemia (CLL).

Chronic Lymphocytic Leukemia (CLL)

CLL is a type of leukemia in which the lymphocytes (white blood cells) begin to grow and change abnormally, preventing the production of oxygen-carrying red blood cells, healthy white blood cells, and platelets. Most often, the disease is diagnosed when too many lymphocytes are found in the blood; however, the same disease can occur when the abnormal lymphocytes are mostly in the lymph nodes but not in the blood. This is called **small lymphocytic lymphoma**, but it is very similar to CLL.

Chronic lymphocytic leukemia is the second most common type of adult leukemia, and is marked by slow progression. Caucasian males, middle-aged or older, bear the highest risk factor, as well as those with a family history of CLL or cancer of the lymph system. Also at higher risk are Russian or Eastern European Jews.

Chronic Myeloid Leukemia (CML)

CML is a slowly progressing form of blood cancer that usually occurs beginning in middle age. Normally, the bone marrow produces stem cells (immature cells) that mature over time. These cells can become either a myeloid cell or a lymphoid cell. In CML, too many myeloid cells become abnormal. These abnormal cells are called "granulocytes."

CML is easy to diagnose because it has a genetic marker, called the "Philadelphia chromosome," named after the city in which it was discovered. This genetic marker occurs by chance, though, and is not passed down from generation to generation.

The classification of leukemia according to type is extremely complex, so a precise diagnosis must be done correctly right from the start in order for the patient to have the best chance for survival. There are also various types of more rare leukemias, such as monocytic leukemia, hairy-cell leukemia, promyelocytic leukemia, erythroleukemia, and others. "Most blood cancers like leukemia are uncommon, and if you go to a community hospital, they are most likely to treat only the most common cancers, so you need to make sure your doctor is either a hematologist (a doctor who specializes in blood diseases) or an oncologist with experience in treating adult leukemia," advises Patrick J. Stiff, MD, hematologist and director of Loyola's Cardinal Bernardin Cancer Center.

"Making an accurate diagnosis and getting the best possible therapy for leukemia is extremely important. There are a lot of nuances in therapy and so it's difficult for a general oncologist, who treats only common cancers like breast or colon cancer, to keep up. It's where you get your first therapy that could determine whether you're cured or not," he adds.

Stages of Leukemia

Leukemia and other blood cancers differ from solid-tumor cancers because the cancerous cells are scattered throughout the body via the bloodstream. Because of the progression of leukemia, most cases are classified according to phases. How the leukemia is treated will depend on the disease's phase.

STAGING AML

AML is divided into eight different subtypes according to the characteristics of the cells and other factors. Treatment and prognosis depends on the subtype of the disease. The vast majority of AML patients require prompt treatment due to the aggressive nature of the disease.

STAGING ALL

ALL is treated according to one's age, condition at diagnosis, and specific results of cellular testing. The term **recent** is used to describe an individual who has been newly diagnosed, while **relapsed** refers to those no longer in remission, or whose condition is recurrent. The objective of ALL treatment is a cure, and it is divided into four stages. Heavy chemotherapy is used during the first two phases, while the third and fourth phases involve maintenance chemotherapies. The entire course of treatment takes between two to three years to complete.

STAGING CML

The three phases of CML are chronic, accelerated, and blast (or blastic).

Chronic Stage
In this initial phase, there are fewer than five percent blast cells, or promyelocytes (immature granulocytes), in the blood and bone marrow. There are only mild symptoms, and conventional treatment is effective.

Accelerated Phase
There are more than five percent but fewer than 30 percent blast cells. The leukemic cells exhibit more chromosomal abnormalities, and so more abnormal cells are produced. Treatment is more intensive.

Blast Phase (Acute Phase, Blast Crisis)
In this final phase, the disease transforms into an aggressive, acute leukemia (either AML or ALL). More than 30 percent of the cells in the blood and bone marrow samples are blast cells, and these cells often invade other tissues and organs. If untreated, this form of CML claims roughly 20 percent of all patients each year.

STAGING CLL
There are five stages of CLL. Each stage is classified according to a scale called the **Rai system** (the Binet system is widely used in Europe), and depends on the amount of lymphocytes in the blood and whether the lymph nodes, spleen, or liver is involved, as well as whether the patient is anemic. Also taken into consideration is whether the blood platelet count is normal or reduced. The Rai system ranges from Stage 0 to IV, with each stage increasing in severity.

Signs and Symptoms
The symptoms of leukemia vary according to type:

AML SYMPTOMS
Early signs of AML can mimic the flu. Symptoms can also include the following:

- Fever
- Bone pain
- Lethargy and fatigue
- Shortness of breath

- Paleness

- Frequent infections

- Easy bruising and unusual bleeding, such as frequent nose-bleeds or bleeding gums

ALL SYMPTOMS

Like AML, early ALL can also produce flu-like symptoms. Additional symptoms are also similar to those of AML.

CML SYMPTOMS

In its early stages, there may be no symptoms, and the disease may be discovered accidentally. Symptoms of advanced CML include the following:

- Unwell appearance

- Fevers

- Bruising easily

- Bone pain

This chronic phase can last from several months to several years.

CLL SYMPTOMS

Usually, CLL does not cause any symptoms and is discovered during a routine blood test. Symptoms are similar to ALL and AML.

The Role of the Spleen

The spleen is an organ in the abdomen that is involved in the production and removal of blood cells. In leukemia, abnormal blood cells form so fast that the spleen can become enlarged.

DID YOU KNOW . . .

Petechiae is the medical term for tiny red or brown spots that may appear on the skin of people with leukemia. They are caused by tiny hemorrhages due to low blood count and the blood's diminished ability to clot.

Specific Diagnostic Tests

A physical examination and blood tests are the first steps used in diagnosing leukemia. If the results of the blood test are not normal, the following tests may be used:

BONE MARROW BIOPSY

For this test, the doctor inserts a long needle into a bone (usually the pelvic bone or breastbone) and then draws out some fluid to analyze the blood cells and see if they are mature or abnormal. If something is wrong, the percentage of abnormal cells is used to classify the leukemia according to type.

CLASSIFICATION TESTS

If leukemia is diagnosed, there are several different methods that can be used to determine its exact type, such as staining the cells, attaching special antibodies to them, or analyzing the antigens (foreign bodies that prompt immune response) they have. These tests are called **cytochemistry**, **flow cytometry**, and **immuno-histochemistry**, respectively.

GENETIC TESTING

Leukemia cells may undergo genetic changes, and recognizing them can help determine both the form of the disease and the most effective treatment. Tests involve studying the cells under the microscope to analyze the DNA and determine whether any abnormal changes have occurred. These tests go by different names, which include **cytogenics, fluorescent in situ hybridization (FISH)**, and **polymerase chain reaction (PCR)**.

LUMBAR PUNCTURE (SPINAL TAP)

This test involves using a hollow needle to remove fluid from the spine. It is performed to see if there are any leukemia cells in the **cerebrospinal fluid (CSF)**, the liquid that surrounds the brain and spinal cord.

IMAGING TESTS

CT (CAT) scans, PET scans, and ultrasound tests can be used to determine if leukemia cells have spread to lymph nodes or organs inside the abdomen, like the kidneys, liver and spleen, or to the bones.

Treatments

The way leukemia is treated differs according to its stage, and whether the disease is acute or chronic. Generally, intensive chemotherapy is used for acute leukemia to cure it, put it into remission, manage the disease, and for use in case of relapse. Chronic leukemia sometimes only needs monitoring in its early stages, and chemotherapy once the condition becomes threatening. Treatments that leukemia patients undergo, especially intensive chemotherapy, and/or bone marrow transplantation, leave the body very vulnerable to infections and lung diseases, so supportive care and strict avoidance of infection are essential.

CHEMOTHERAPY

Chemotherapy is a mainstay in the treatment of leukemia. In fact, **imatinib (Gleevec)**, a chemotherapy drug that dates back a half century, is credited with the turnaround in leukemia survival rates. Gleevec received FDA approval in 2001, made the cover of *Time* magazine the following year, and has been hailed for transforming leukemia from a potentially fatal disease to a chronic, manageable one. It is a first-line therapy for acute and chronic leukemia patients, and used at higher dosages for bone marrow transplants recipients.

IMMUNOTHERAPY

In 2014, the FDA approved Blinocyto (blinatumomab), an immunological agent to treat a rare form of ALL known as "**Philadelphia chromosome-negative precursor B-cell acute lymhoblastic leukemia,**" or B-cell ALL.

GOOD ADVICE

If you are a Vietnam War veteran who was exposed to Agent Orange during the war and you've been diagnosed with leukemia, you may (depending on the type) qualify for VA disability compensation and special access to medical care. See the appendix for more information.

SPLENECTOMY

This surgery is not usually needed, but is performed when the disease has caused the organ to enlarge and is pressing on other organs, or it is turning out too many abnormal white cells, depriving the body of red blood cells and/or or platelets. Most live very well without a spleen, but it does increase the risk of infections. In some cases, radiation is done to shrink the spleen.

BONE MARROW TRANSPLANTS

A bone marrow transplant can be done in severe cases of adult leukemia and non-Hodgkin's lymphoma. This procedure replaces damaged or destroyed marrow with healthy marrow stem cells.

13

Melanoma

DARYN MAYER WAS 29 when she first noticed an odd-looking freckle on her thigh. "I had lots of freckles, but this one looked different," says Mayer, who is now 42. She went to a dermatologist, but he seemed more interested in selling her skin products. He told her the freckle was nothing to worry about, but, as she watched it grow and change color, she grew more and more worried. Finally, she called the doctor again and was offered an appointment two months away. "I really need this looked at. I am coming to the office today and I will sit there until I'm seen." This time, the doctor took her concerns seriously, and performed a biopsy. The "freckle" turned out to be a melanoma. But it was caught early, thanks to Mayer's insistence, and today, many years later, she remains cancer-free.

What Is Melanoma?

Melanoma arises from the skin, which is our body's largest organ. The skin is made up of two main layers, the outer, **epidermis**, and the inner, **dermis**. There is also a deeper third layer with cells called melanocytes. These cells produce melanin, the dark pigment from which melanoma develops. Commonly melanoma develops in the skin. It can also develop in the colon or within the white lining of the eye; both these forms are very rare.

Statistics

Melanoma accounts for just a tiny percentage of skin cancer cases, but it causes the majority of skin cancer deaths. Approximately 80,000 new melanomas will be diagnosed (roughly 45,000 men and 35,000 women). About 9,500 people die of melanoma each year (about 6,500 men and 3,000 women).

The rates of skin cancer have skyrocketed over the past decades, and this includes melanoma. "The incidence of melanoma has increased 200 percent over the past 30 years, which is alarming," says skin care specialist Alysa Herman, MD, citing a Skin Cancer Foundation report.

The risk of melanoma increases with age because damage to skin accumulates over the years. The average age at the time of diagnosis is 63 for men and 56 for women. More women than men are diagnosed with melanoma prior to the age of 40 and after that, the gender balance switches. The survival rate is also higher in women than it is in men.

Although melanoma is rare before age 30, in those aged 20 to 29 years it is the third most commonly diagnosed cancer after thyroid and testicular cancer, and its incidence is climbing, especially in young women.

Caucasians are far more likely than African-Americans to develop melanoma, especially those with light skin, light hair, and freckles. Scientists recently discovered a genetic link between melanoma and people with red hair. Although melanoma mainly develops in Caucasians, people who are African-American are vulnerable to a rare form of melanoma. This form of occurs in the areas of lighter skin not usually exposed to the sun, such as the palms of the hands, the soles of the feet, under fingernails, and in the mouth.

Like other cancers, melanoma is influenced by genetics. About 10 percent of people with melanoma have family members who have had the disease. There are certain genetic disorders that greatly increase the risk for melanoma. These include **dysplastic nevus mole syndrome** (*nevus* comes from the Latin for "mole") and **FAM-M, familial atypical multiple mose melanoma syndrome**. FAM-M raises the risk for a number of cancers, including those of the eye, breast, respiratory tract, gastrointestinal tract, and the lymphatic system.

You are most likely to develop inherited melanoma if you have a close relative with it, or if you were born with atypical moles. Sun exposure plays a role, but the link is weaker here. "It's not that the sun is not responsible for contributing to melanoma, it's just that the effect is not as high as for other forms of skin cancer," Dr. Herman says. She's very much concerned about the rise in popularity of indoor tanning beds. "It's been found that just one indoor tanning session raises melanoma risk by 20 percent. This is of huge importance," she adds.

There is a link between melanoma and breast and prostate cancer. Doctors should warn patients with either breast cancer or melanoma that they should be monitored for the other cancer as well. This is also true of prostate cancer. Researchers recently found that men with prostate cancer are at a roughly twofold increased risk for melanoma.

Outcome and Survival Rates

There are nearly a million melanoma survivors living in the United States today (roughly 481,000 men and 496,000 women). "The good news is that survival rates are up. In the early 1950s, there was a 49 percent survival rate, which has increased to an overall 92 percent rate today," says Dr. Herman.

When diagnosed in its earliest stages, melanoma has a 99 percent cure rate, while the survival rate for Stage IV melanomas in which the cancer has spread to distant organs drops to 15 to 20 percent. However, Stages II and III are subdivided into categories that overlap, meaning that some Stage III melanomas are less dangerous than Stage II. (See the section on staging for more information.)

"When it comes to cancer, making survival predictions is difficult, but this is especially true when it comes to melanoma. With all of the research we've done, this is the one type of cancer that's eluded us in terms of its molecular biology. We can't predict the people who will develop it, or those who will survive it," Dr. Herman says.

The Four Types of Melanoma

SUPERFICIAL SPREADING MELANOMA

This type of melanoma is the most common type and accounts for around 70 percent of cases. It generally appears as a flat or slightly raised discolored patch with irregular borders. It occurs more commonly in women and can develop from a mole. It can arise anywhere, but usually appears on the trunk in men, the legs in women, and the upper back of both genders.

NODULAR MELANOMA

This rare, fast-spreading melanoma usually occurs in men. The moles appear suddenly and may resemble blood blisters, although they may range in color from blue-black to white and include a variety of hues including tan, brown, and red.

LENTIGO MALIGNA MELANOMA

Occurring most often in people over 50, these moles usually appear on the face, ears, neck, or other parts of the body that have received long-term sun exposure. This type is also known as **Hutchinson's melanotic freckle**, affecting those who have been exposed to the sun for years.

ACRAL LENTIGINOUS MELANOMA

This type of melanoma appears as a black or brown discoloration, often on the palms of the hands and the soles of the feet. It occurs most often in African-Americans and Asians.

Stages of Melanoma

The staging system for melanoma is extremely complicated. Two staging systems are used — **Breslow's classification**, which looks at the vertical thickness in millimeters, or **Clark's classification**, which takes into consideration the level of the tumor.

Each stage of melanoma is determined by several characteristics, including how widespread and thick the abnormality is, whether it is ulcerated, how fast its cells are dividing, and whether it has spread to the lymph nodes or other organs in the body, among other characteristics.

STAGE 0

This is a situation in which abnormal melanocytes are found in the upper layer of the skin (epidermis) but have not reached the second layer (dermis). Stage 0 is also called melanoma in situ.

STAGE I

This stage is divided into the following two categories:

Stage IA: The tumor is less than or equal to one millimeter (mm) with no ulceration.

Stage IB: The tumor is no more than one mm, with ulceration, or the tumor is between one and two mm, without ulceration.

STAGE II

This stage is divided into the following three categories:

Stage IIA: The melanoma is between one mm and two mm in thickness and is ulcerated, or it is between two and four mm and is not ulcerated.

Stage IIB: The melanoma is between two mm and four mm in thickness and is ulcerated, or it is thicker than four mm and is not ulcerated.

Stage IIC: The melanoma is more than four mm in thickness and is ulcerated, or it is thicker than four mm and is not ulcerated.

STAGE III

In Stage III, one of the three situations apply:

Stage IIIA: The melanoma can be of any thickness and is ulcerated. It has spread to one to three lymph nodes near the affected skin area. The nodes are enlarged because of the melanoma. There is no distant spread.

Stage IIIB: The melanoma can be of any thickness and is ulcerated. It has spread to small areas of nearby skin or lymphatic channels around the original tumor, but the nodes do not contain melanoma. There is no distant spread.

Stage IIIC: The melanoma can be of any thickness and may or may not be ulcerated. It has spread to four or more nearby lymph nodes, or to nearby lymph nodes that are clumped together, or it has spread to nearby skin or lymphatic channels around the original tumor and to nearby lymph nodes. The nodes are enlarged because of the melanoma. There is no distant spread.

STAGE IV

The melanoma has spread beyond the original area of skin and nearby lymph nodes to other organs such as the lung, liver, or brain, or to distant areas of the skin, subcutaneous tissue, or distant lymph nodes. Neither spread to nearby lymph nodes nor thickness is considered in this stage, but typically the melanoma is thick and has also spread to the lymph nodes.

Signs and Symptoms

The signs and symptoms of melanoma change as the disease progresses.

EARLY WARNING SIGNS
Moles

The single early warning sign of melanoma is a change in a mole or skin growth. Virtually all light-skinned people are born with a few moles, and they can change as we age. Not all moles are potentially dangerous, but new moles that appear in adults or mole changes should be checked. Here are the **ABCDEs** that indicate suspicious moles:

- **A**symmetry: An "atypical" mole is asymmetrical, which means it is irregular in shape. In other words, if you draw an imaginary line through it, you would not have matching halves. Such a mole can be a sign of trouble.

- **B**order: The borders of early melanomas are usually uneven, containing scalloped or notched edges.

- **C**olor: Moles are usually a single shade of brown, so a mole with different shades of brown or black may be the first sign of melanoma. Also, beware of moles that lose color or turn white.

- **D**iameter: Most harmless moles are usually less than one-quarter inch in diameter — the size of a pencil eraser. Early melanomas tend to be larger than this.

- **E**volving: Any change — in size, shape, color, elevation, or another trait, or any new symptom such as bleeding, itching, or crusting — points to danger.

Additional Signs and Symptoms:
- Changes in the surface of the mole, such as it becoming scaly, oozing, bleeding, or the appearance of a bump or nodule

- A sore that does not heal

- Spread of pigment from the border of a spot to surrounding skin

- Redness or a new swelling beyond the border

- Change in sensation — itchiness, tenderness, or pain

GOOD ADVICE

Seborrheic keratosis (noncancerous skin growths that come with aging), warts, and basal cell cancer (a less serious form of skin cancer) can look similar to melanoma, but don't attempt to diagnose your moles and skin changes yourself — see a dermatologist.

Specific Diagnostic Tests
PHYSICAL EXAMINATION

The doctor does an overall check of the skin and also makes note of any moles so they can be tracked for changes over time. If any suspicious moles or skin growths are seen, the next step is a biopsy.

BIOPSY

A biopsy involves taking a sample of skin from a suspicious area to be examined under a microscope. There are several different types of biopsies that can be preformed, depending on the size of the affected area, where it is located on the body, and other factors. Any biopsy can leave a small scar, so if the affected area is on the face, or other area you are concerned about, ask your doctor about it. Here's a rundown on different types of biopsies that can be done:

- **Skin biopsy:** A sample of skin is taken and sent to the pathologist to be examined under a microscope.

- **Shave biopsy:** The top layers of skin are shaved off with a small surgical blade.

- **Punch biopsy:** An instrument that looks like a tiny round cookie cutter is used to cut through several layers of skin. This type of biopsy usually requires stitches.

- **Incisional and excisional biopsies:** A surgical knife is used to cut through all the layers of the skin in order to take a sample, or to completely remove a melanoma if possible.

DIAGNOSTIC TESTS TO FIND OUT IF MELANOMA HAS SPREAD

Melanoma is spread through the body's lymph system. If a diagnosis of melanoma is confirmed, here are the tests used to find out if it may have spread:

Lymph Node Biopsy

A lymph node or a piece of a lymph node is removed for examination under a microscope. This can be done in the following ways:

- **Fine needle aspiration biopsy:** A syringe with a thin hollow needle is used to biopsy the lymph nodes to find out if a melanoma has spread to them.

- **Surgical (excisional) lymph node biopsy:** An enlarged lymph node is removed through a small incision in the skin.

- **Sentinel lymph node biopsy:** This test is used to see if melanoma has spread to nearby lymph nodes and to stage the tumor. The test is conducted by the use of a small amount of radioactive substance, or blue dye, which is injected into the area of the melanoma. Then the lymph nodes are checked to see if the substance has spread to them. If no melanoma cells are found, no additional surgery is needed because the melanoma is unlikely to have spread. A lymph node dissection (lymphadenectomy) used to be done for diagnostic purposes to see if the melanoma had spread to the lymph nodes, but the sentinel lymph node biopsy has replaced this, so that no lymph nodes are needlessly removed, which can cause complications.

IMAGING TESTS

In melanoma, as with other cancers, a variety of imaging tests can be used to see if the tumor has spread to other organs in the body. They include chest X-ray, CT (CAT), MRI and PET scans.

MOLECULAR TESTING

Molecular tests are performed on the tumor in order to find genetic factors that can help determine treatment. In the case of melanoma, 40 to 60 percent of tumors have a defect in the **BRAF** gene, a human gene that makes a protein called B-Raf.

Treatments

As with other types of cancer, the treatment for melanoma depends on the location, extent, and stage of the tumor. In early-stage melanoma, the primary treatment is surgery. In the later stages, surgery is often used in combination with other treatments including chemotherapy, radiation, and targeted therapy as well.

> **GOOD ADVICE**
>
> Melanoma can be difficult to classify and stage properly, but treatment depends on this being done correctly right from the start. So make sure that your biopsy results are read by an experienced dermatopathologist, who is a pathologist specializing in skin diseases.

SURGERY

Simple Excision

If the suspicious lesion or tissue abnormality is thin, it can be removed by a minor operation called a skin excision. The tumor is simply cut out and then stitched closed. Early melanomas can be cured with this procedure.

Wide Excision

If the biopsy confirms the suspicious lesion is melanoma, the area will need to be reopened and more skin cut away and examined under a microscope to make sure that no cancer cells are left in the skin.

Mohs Surgery

This is a type of skin surgery that can be done in place of a wide excision when the tumor appears on the face. This micrographic procedure involves removing tissue and checking it under a microscope during the surgery to ensure that only the cancerous tissue is removed. This allows for the preservation of healthy skin, which makes for the best cosmetic effect. An experienced skin cancer surgeon should be chosen for this procedure.

Lymphadenectomy (Lymph Node Dissection/Removal)

This is the procedure that may be done if the sentinel lymph node biopsy shows that the cancer has spread to the lymph nodes. Removing the lymph nodes is a serious procedure, because this is the body's drainage system that prevents fluid from collecting in the arms and legs (a condition called lymphedema), so the doctor will not do it unless it is deemed necessary.

Surgery for Advanced Melanoma

When the melanoma has spread from the skin to distant organs (such as the lungs or brain), the cancer is very unlikely to be cured by surgery. Even so, surgery is sometimes done because removing even a few areas of spread could help some people to live longer or have a better quality of life. If you have metastatic melanoma and your doctor recommends surgery, be sure you understand what the goal of the surgery would be.

CHEMOTHERAPY

Chemical treatment is usually not as effective on melanoma as it is for other types of cancer; however, it is often used around the lymph nodes when they are removed, or if the cancer is on the arms or legs. In this procedure, blood flow to rest of the body is temporarily stopped so the anticancer drugs can be infused directly into the affected limb at higher doses than ordinarily performed.

RADIATION

Radiation is sometimes used on other organs to which the melanoma has spread, like the bone or brain, to help shrink the tumor and relieve symptoms.

IMMUNOTHERAPY

Immunologic drugs are getting much attention in the treatment of advanced melanoma. These include the cytokines **interferon** and **interleukin-2 (IL-2)**, which act as proteins to boost the immune system. Other agents are **pembrolizumab**

(Keytruda), **nivolumab (Opdivo)**, and **ipilimumab (Yervoy)**. The bacillus Calmette-Guérin (BCG) vaccine is also used to bolster the immune system.

TARGETED THERAPY

Targeted therapy, known also as **personalized therapy** or **molecular therapies**, is one of the most promising methods currently used to treat melanoma. This involves the use of drugs that are "targeted" through genetics and other factors, and can destroy cancer cells while leaving normal cells intact.

An estimated 50 percent of people with melanoma have changes in the BRAF protein. The BRAF protein is part of the MAP kinase pathway — a chain of enzymatic reactions that include the enzyme MEK, which becomes overactive and enables the cancer to grow. These particular drugs will only work on tumors with the BRAF protein. They are effective, though, and since melanoma is so hard to treat, this shows why these tumors must be genetically analyzed.

Here's a rundown on the targeted drugs currently in use:

- **Zelboraf (vemurafenib)** is approved for the treatment of BRAF V600E mutant melanoma that cannot be removed by surgery. This drug is only approved for those patients who have tested positive for the BRAF mutation.

- **Tafinlar (dabrafenib)** is approved to treat of BRAF V600 mutant melanoma that cannot be removed by surgery. This drug is only approved for those patients who have tested positive for the BRAF mutation and is not indicated for patients with wild-type BRAF mutation.

- **Mekinist (trametinib)** is approved for BRAF V600E or V600K mutations. It is a first-class MEK inhibitor approved for the treatment of unresectable or metastatic melanoma, and cannot be used on patients who have undergone BRAF inhibitor therapy.

GOOD ADVICE

Melanoma survivors are at higher risk of developing additional melanomas, so sun protection is a must! Avoid the hours when the sun is most intense (10 a.m. to 2 p.m.). Wear sunscreen with high SPF and sun-protective clothing.

Non-Hodgkin's Lymphoma

14

JOY HUBER WAS 33, single, had just sold her house and was in the middle of packing up to move to Nashville in pursuit of her dream as a songwriter when she was diagnosed with non-Hodgkin's lymphoma. "Lymph node cancer? Not at 33! I remember standing in my bathroom, looking in the mirror at my reflection, saying, 'You have cancer. YOU have cancer . . . YOU HAVE CAN-CER!' But I still could not completely wrap my mind around it," she recalls.

But, indeed, Huber did have Stage IV follicular lymphoma, a slowly progressing form of non-Hodgkin's lymphoma that, although treatable, is difficult to cure. She underwent intensive chemotherapy and, now in remission, strives to help others as an author and speaker, spreading awareness.

What Is Non-Hodgkin's Lymphoma?

Lymph is a clear fluid that circulates through the body via a channel called the lymph system. One of its main functions is to rid the body of toxins as part of our immune defense. Non-Hodgkin's lymphoma begins when certain cells in the lymphatic system change and begin to grow uncontrollably, which may form a tumor. Non-Hodgkin's lymphoma is the overall term for a large, diverse group of cancers.

Statistics

Each year, an estimated 70,000 people (37,000 men and 33,000 women) are diagnosed with non-Hodgkin's lymphoma. Most people develop the disease for no known reason, but growing older heightens risk. The most common forms of non-Hodgkin's lymphoma occur in those between ages 60 and 70, but people of any age can develop it. The disease is also more common in men.

"Often, when non-Hodgkin's lymphoma appears in younger people, the course of the disease is more aggressive than in people who are older and usually have the slower growing, indolent types," says Dr. Alexandra Stefanovic, a hematological oncologist with the Sylvester Comprehensive Cancer Center at the University of Miami. "The number of cases of non-Hodgkin's lymphoma has been increasing since the 1970s, although it isn't completely understood why," Dr. Stefanovic adds.

Factors that affect the immune system can raise the risk for non-Hodgkin's lymphoma. These include bacterial infections, such as the bacterium *Helicobacter pylori*, which also causes stomach ulcers. Viruses such as **Epstein-Barr** that causes mononucleosis, is associated with some types of non-Hodgkin's lymphoma, as well as hepatitis C.

Immune deficiency disorders, such as HIV/AIDS, greatly hike the risk of this disease. People with autoimmune disorders, such as rheumatoid arthritis and Sjögren's syndrome, are also at higher risk, although to a far lesser extent. Another high-risk group is people who have undergone organ (kidney, liver, heart, or lung) transplantation, because of the drugs they must take to prevent organ rejection.

There are genetic factors that involve DNA, but they are not of the same types that occur in many other forms of cancer. In some other types of cancer, hereditary factors can play a role, at least in terms of making people more prone to develop the disease if their parents or close relatives are affected. This is not the case with non-Hodgkin's lymphoma. Although changes in a patient's DNA do occur, these changes occur after birth. Such acquired changes can occur with exposure to the factors cited above, as well as to radiation and cancer-causing chemicals, like pesticides and petrochemicals, or such mutations can occur for no known reason.

Outcome and Survival Rates

There are about 535,000 non-Hodgkin's lymphoma survivors in the United States today. This tally includes 280,000 men and 255,000 women.

Non-Hodgkin's lymphoma is one of the more curable types of cancer. The one-year relative survival rate is 81 percent. The five-year and 10-year relative survival rates are 68 percent and 57 percent, respectively. It is estimated that 19,000 (10,600 men and 8,400 women) deaths from this disease occur each year.

Although there is still work to be done, the cure rate for non-Hodgkin's lymphoma has risen dramatically over the years. This success stems from an increased understanding of the disease, coupled with the development of better treatments that have improved outcomes. "The five-year survival rate for patients with non-Hodgkin's lymphoma has probably doubled over the last several years," says Dr. Patrick Stiff.

One of the factors that revolutionized the treatment of non-Hodgkin's lymphoma was the development of the drug **rituximab (Rituxan)**, which is a monoclonal antibody that targets a protein found on the surface of immune system B cells and acts to destroy them. Most types of non-Hodgkin's lymphoma are characterized by an excessive number of B cells, overactive B cells, or dysfunctional B cells.

Another reason why non-Hodgkin's lymphoma is more easily treated than some other forms of cancer is that lymphomas are generally very sensitive to chemotherapy and radiation and, unlike most other cancers, do not require surgery.

GOOD ADVICE

Because such a large percentage of patients with non-Hodgkin's lymphoma live many years after treatment, it is essential to find a doctor with whom you can form a relationship, not only during your treatment, but also for many years to come.

Types of Non-Hodgkin's Lymphoma

Non-Hodgkin's lymphoma is an overall term for a type of cancer that takes many different forms, and which can require different types of care and treatment.

There are so many different types of lymphoma that it's really a large family of diseases with many different characteristics. "In fact, the disease is so individualized that it's almost impossible to draw generalizations from one case to another," Dr. Stefanovic says.

This is why patients who are newly diagnosed with non-Hodgkin's lymphoma must seek out a specialist with extensive experience in treating the disease. "Lymphomas are of such different types, and there are so many differences being discovered between all the different subtypes and their response to treatment, that it is difficult for anyone who is not a lymphoma expert to keep up," she notes.

There are three major groups of lymphoma and they are classified by the type of immune cell in which the disease began:

B-CELL LYMPHOMA

This is the most common type of non-Hodgkin's lymphoma and accounts for about 85 percent of the cases.

T-CELL LYMPHOMA

This type of lymphoma occurs in less than 15 percent of cases.

NK-CELL LYMPHOMA

This is rare form of non-Hodgkin's lymphoma that accounts for about one percent of cases. NK, which stands for "natural killer" cell, has caused much controversy regarding its classification. The jury is still out as to whether this is a T-cell lymphoma with abnormal markers, or if these destructive cells do, in fact, belong in a class of their own.

NON-HODGKIN'S LYMPHOMA SUBGROUPS

There are also many different subgroups of non-Hodgkin's lymphoma. Many are rare, but here are the two most common:

Diffuse Large B-Cell Lymphoma (DLBCL)

This type accounts for about 30 percent of cases. It is an aggressive form of non-Hodgkin's lymphoma that spreads to other organs about 40 percent of the time.

Other (aggressive) types of non-Hodgkin's lymphoma, which are rarer, include the following:

- Peripheral T-cell lymphoma

- Burkitt's lymphoma

- Anaplastic large cell lymphoma

- Lymphoblastic lymphoma

Follicular Lymphoma

This slow-growing (indolent) form of non-Hodgkin's lymphoma accounts for 20 percent of the cases. Although not curable, this form of non-Hodgkin's lymphoma grows so slowly that 50 percent of those with it live at least 12 more years, and many longer. For some patients, "watchful waiting," or monitoring, is the sole treatment. In other cases, treatment with a combination of chemotherapy, targeted therapies, monoclonal antibodies (a type of targeted therapy), and/or radiation is required. Sometimes, these slow-growing lymphomas can change into more aggressive types. When that happens, they require aggressive treatment.

Other subtypes of indolent lymphoma include **Small lymphocytic lymphoma**, which is the same as **chronic lymphocytic leukemia (CLL)**, **marginal zone lymphoma/MALT lymphoma**, and **mantle cell lymphoma**. For more on CLL, see the chapter on leukemia.

ADDITIONAL RARE TYPES OF NON-HODGKIN'S LYMPHOMA

- **MALT lymphoma:** Muscosa associated lymphoid tissue is a B-cell lymphoma that starts in the lining of other organs. MALT lymphoma is most common in the stomach. It is linked to bacterial infection with *Helicobacter pylori* and can be treated with antibiotics.

- **Mantle cell lymphoma:** This type of NHL is a B-cell lymphoma, which occurs most often in men over the age of 50. Although classified as low-grade, mantle cell often behaves aggressively and so is treated as such.

GOOD ADVICE

Non-Hodgkin's lymphoma is so complex that choosing a doctor who is highly experienced, such as a hematological oncologist (blood cancer specialist), is essential right from the start. "When it comes to non-Hodgkin's lymphoma, there are a lot of nuances, so if the initial treatment is wrong, the patient may be led down the wrong path. It's where you get your first therapy that determines cure or no cure," says Dr. Stiff.

Stages of Non-Hodgkin's Lymphoma

The traditional staging system used for most cancers is not used for non-Hodgkin's lymphoma. Instead, the main types of non-Hodgkin's lymphoma are grouped from low-grade (indolent) to high-grade (aggressive). They are characterized according to how quickly they spread as well as the tumor cell's shape and size. In addition, these classifications are divided into two subtypes, and labeled A and B based on the person's symptoms. "A" means the person has **not** experienced the following, "B" symptoms:

- Unexplained weight loss of 10 percent within six months before diagnosis
- Unexplained fever
- Drenching sweats during the night (most commonly) or daytime

Signs and Symptoms

- A painless lump in the neck, armpit, or groin
- An enlarged liver or spleen
- Shortness of breath
- Fever
- Sweating and chills
- Fatigue

Specific Diagnostic Tests

PHYSICAL EXAMINATION

The doctor performs a physical examination, paying special attention to the lymph nodes, liver, and spleen.

BIOPSY

A small amount of tissue is removed, usually from the lymph nodes in the neck, under an arm, or in the groin, and examined under a microscope. In some cases, a biopsy may be taken from the chest or abdomen during a computed tomography (CT scan) or by using an endoscope (a thin, lighted, flexible tube) to take a sample from the stomach or intestine.

IMAGING TESTS

A variety of imaging tests, including CT, MRI, and PET scans, can be used to detect any spread of the cancer.

BONE MARROW BIOPSY AND ASPIRATION

Lymphoma often spreads to the bone marrow. This test is important for both obtaining diagnostic information and staging the disease.

MOLECULAR TESTING

Once a diagnosis of non-Hodgkin's lymphoma is confirmed, specific tests are performed on the lymphoma cells to identify specific genes, proteins, chromosome changes, and other factors unique to the disease to determine the most effective treatment.

Treatments

The treatment for non-Hodgkin's lymphoma depends on whether the type is indolent (slow growing), aggressive (fast growing), and where exactly it falls along this scale.

Also, unlike most cancers, which are solid tumors, non-Hodgkin's lymphoma is a blood cancer, so instead of surgery, the general treatment is usually a combination of chemotherapy and immunological treatments involving monoclonal antibodies (a type of biological treatment). If the disease is severe and aggressive, a bone marrow transplant may be recommended to enable the patient to withstand high doses of chemotherapy.

The following is a description of treatments according to non-Hodgkin's lymphoma type:

- **Diffuse large B-cell lymphoma (DLBCL):** In forms of aggressive non-Hodgkin's lymphoma, the basis for curing or bringing about remission is the administration of chemotherapy drugs, most notably a combination of four drugs that go by the acronym of **CHOP: cyclophosphamide, doxorubicin, vincristine,** and **prednisone.** Rituxan (rituximab), which is a targeted biological agent that kills cancer cells, is also often used, and radiation can be added if the lymphoma is in a small, localized area. Different chemotherapy regimens can be used if the cancer returns.

• **Follicular lymphoma:** This is a slow-growing lymphoma that is very treatable but difficult to cure. Treatment depends on several factors. Sometimes, no treatment is recommended until or if symptoms appear. Then, treatment depends on the stage. Treatments can range from radiation, the administration of Rituxan alone or combined with chemotherapy, or the four-drug CHOP regimen. Radioactive monoclonal antibodies are also treatment options, either used alone or in combination with chemotherapy.

STEM CELL TRANSPLANT

A stem cell transplant is sometimes used to treat non-Hodgkin's lymphoma as a means of curing the disease, or if it returns after remission. This is an intensive procedure that allows doctors to administer higher doses of chemotherapy than would otherwise be tolerated. See chapter 3 for more information.

BONE MARROW TRANSPLANT

Like a stem cell transplant, a bone marrow transplant (from a related or unrelated donor) also enables the administration of high-dose chemotherapy. This treatment is generally reserved for younger patients who are in otherwise good health, and for whom conventional treatments would not result in a cure.

GOOD ADVICE

While it's tempting to listen to other patients' stories, don't fall into the trap of comparing your treatment to theirs. "These cancers are very individualized, so if someone tells you they had non-Hodgkin's lymphoma and X, Y, and Z was done to treat it, don't compare your own treatment. No treatment is exactly the same, so what worked for one person won't necessarily apply to you."
—Dr. Stefanovic

Ovarian Cancer

15

GINNY DIXON WAS JUST 31 when was she was diagnosed with ovarian cancer. Her periods stopped and her doctor was trying hormone treatments to correct the problem, but nothing worked. Dixon had no pain or other problems, and, she says, "I forgot about it," until she suddenly began to lose weight. She could see the outline of a bump on her abdomen. Her doctor assumed it was a cyst, but just as Dixon was about to undergo surgery to remove it, her preliminary blood tests showed elevated cancer markers. She underwent surgery, along with very aggressive therapy, and now, some 21 years later, she still considers herself lucky, indeed, to have survived this dangerous type of women's cancer.

What Is Ovarian Cancer?

Ovarian cancer develops in the almond-shaped glands known as the ovaries, which are part of the female reproductive system and situated on either side of the uterus. They produce egg cells (ova), and also provide the main source of the female hormones, which govern the development of female characteristics, including breasts, body shape and body hair, as well as the female reproductive cycle.

Statistics

Each year, more than 22,000 women in the United States are diagnosed with ovarian cancer — the eighth most common cancer (excluding skin cancer), and the fifth leading cause of cancer in women. In all, ovarian cancer constitutes 1.3 percent of all newly diagnosed cancer cases this year.

Any women without risk factors can develop ovarian cancer. Genetics do play a role, as women with a family history of ovarian cancer are at higher risk, and this is also true for those with a personal or family history of breast cancer.

"Genetic factors are linked to about 15 percent of ovarian cancer cases, and those are the only ones that we can detect. The rest are sporadic," says Dr. Stacey Akers, a gynecologic oncologist and assistant professor of oncology at Roswell Park Cancer Institute in Buffalo, New York. "Sporadic" means that the cancer occurs for no known reason.

Caucasians are more likely to develop ovarian cancer, especially those of Jewish Ashkenazi (Eastern European) background. This heritage makes them more likely to have the BRCA1 and BRCA1 genetic mutations.

HNPCC, or Lynch syndrome (see chapter 8), raises ovarian cancer risk, along with uterine, stomach, and kidney cancer.

Hormonal and other factors play a tiny role, too. Infertile women, those who have never become pregnant, or those who first gave birth after the age of 35 are also at slightly higher risk. There was a concern that using fertility drugs heightened risk, but research findings are contradictory. The use of talcum powder in the genital area also has long been suspected, but no link has been proven.

Outcome and Survival Rates

There are nearly 200,000 women in the United States today who are ovarian cancer survivors.

GOOD ADVICE

If you have been diagnosed with ovarian cancer you should seek out genetic counseling to find if heredity played a role in your disease. If you learn that this is the case, you will also have the opportunity to alert your female relatives that they should be evaluated for a screening program. Remember, especially when it comes to ovarian cancer, that early diagnosis saves lives!

As with most other cancer, the earlier the cancer is diagnosed and treated, the higher the survival rate. The overall, five-year survival rate for ovarian cancer is 44 percent, but this varies widely depending on the extent (stage) of the cancer. If the cancer is diagnosed and treated before it has spread outside the ovaries, the five-year survival rate is 92 percent. If the cancer has spread to the surrounding organs or tissue (regional spread), the five-year survival rate is 72 percent. If the cancer has spread to parts of the body far away from the ovary (distant spread), the five-year survival rate falls to 27 percent. These statistics apply specifically to epithelial cancer, which accounts for up to 90 percent of cases.

The main reason why the mortality rate is higher than some other forms of cancer is because this disease can become very advanced before it causes anything but the vaguest of symptoms. Because the ovaries are located in the roomy pelvic cavity, an ovary can balloon to the size of a grapefruit before creating enough pressure to signal a problem. So, by the time ovarian cancer is diagnosed, it may have spread outside the pelvic region, making treatment much more difficult.

The good news, though, is that more women are surviving than ever before. In fact, 44 percent of women with ovarian cancer survive at least five years, and, according to a new survey, one-third was alive after 10 years, including some with high-risk cancers. This is a dramatic increase from 30 years ago, when the five-year survival rate was 10 to 15 percent.

Because ovarian cancer mortality rates are so high, this is a cancer that must be diagnosed, staged, and treated absolutely correctly right from the very beginning — there is no room for error.

"Too often, women are inclined to put their trust in their gynecologist or general surgeon, but a woman with ovarian cancer should be treated by a gynecologic oncologist, right from the start," says Dr. Akers. "This means seeking treatment from a doctor who specializes in the treatment of women with reproductive system cancers."

In addition, the doctor should have treated a lot of ovarian cancer patients. Since ovarian cancer is so deadly, doctors of this type are found at top cancer centers or large medical centers.

Also, ovarian cancer has a high rate of recurrence, so you need an experienced doctor who not only can deal with the disease the first time around, but also can effectively treat it should it return.

Types of Ovarian Cancer

EPITHELIAL CARCINOMA

This cancer, which develops from the cells that line the ovaries, is by far the most common type of ovarian cancer, and accounts for 85 to 90 percent of cases. Half of all cases of epithelial carcinoma occur in women over the age of 65.

DID YOU KNOW . . .

Ovarian cysts are fluid-filled sacs that develop on the outside of the ovary. They are not cancer. They are benign growths that are common, and which most women experience in the course of their lives. Most ovarian cysts disappear within a few months, although some may grow large and need to be removed.

OVARIAN GERM CELL TUMORS

These develop from the cells that produce the ova (the eggs). This is a more rare form of ovarian cancer that occurs in young women. It has a 90 percent cure rate.

LOW MALIGNANT-POTENTIAL OVARIAN TUMORS

LMPs are ovarian epithelial tumors whose appearance under the microscope does not clearly identify them as cancerous. These are called borderline tumors or tumors of low malignant potential.

OVARIAN STROMAL TUMORS

These exceedingly rare tumors develop from connective tissue cells that hold the ovary together and those that produce the female hormones, estrogen and progesterone.

Stages of Ovarian Cancer

Each stage of ovarian cancer has several sub-classifications, but these are the main stages:

STAGE I

The cancer is limited to one or both ovaries.

STAGE II

The cancer is confined to the pelvis.

STAGE III

The disease has spread outside of the pelvis, but is limited to the abdomen, or lymph node involvement.

STAGE IV

The disease spread to the liver or outside of the abdomen.

Signs and Symptoms

The following symptoms may indicate ovarian cancer:

- Abdominal bloating
- Pelvic or abdominal pain
- Difficulty eating or feeling full quickly
- Urinary symptoms (urgency or frequency)
- Fatigue
- Indigestion
- Back pain
- Pain with intercourse
- Constipation
- Menstrual irregularities

The symptoms of ovarian cancer can be vague and be mistaken for lesser problems, like the flu. But it's been found that the first four symptoms on the above list are the ones that occur most often in ovarian cancer. This is why the Ovarian Cancer National Alliance, along with other women's health organizations, urges women to specifically bring up the possibility of cancer with their doctors if the following four symptoms persist longer than two weeks:

- Abdominal bloating
- Pelvic or abdominal pain
- Difficulty eating or feeling full quickly
- Urinary symptoms (urgency or frequency)

GOOD ADVICE

The staging of ovarian cancer is very important. Ovarian cancers not only have different prognoses according to their stage, but they also require different treatment, which impacts survival. So, this is why a gynecological oncologist should perform whatever surgery is necessary right from the very beginning.

Specific Diagnostic Tests

PELVIC EXAM

The doctor feels the uterus, vagina, ovaries, fallopian tubes, bladder, and rectum to check for any unusual changes.

TRANSVAGINAL ULTRASOUND

An ultrasound wand is inserted in the vagina and sound waves are used to create images of the ovaries, including healthy tissues, cysts, and tumors.

CA-125 TEST

This blood test measures a substance called CA-125 in the blood, which is a tumor marker that is found at elevated levels in women with ovarian cancer. It is also used to monitor the effectiveness of treatment. The other tumor marker tests, HE4 and OVA-1, can also aid in diagnosis.

BIOPSY

If these preliminary tests cited above indicate ovarian cancer may be present, a biopsy will be needed to confirm it. This is the removal of tissue for analysis; however, ovarian cancer is different from most other cancers in that a biopsy is rarely done separately. If ovarian cancer is found, surgery will be performed at the same time to remove as much of the tumor as possible. This is the reason why this procedure should be performed by a gynecological oncologist. What happens at this step may determine all future treatment, and could directly impact survival.

GOOD ADVICE

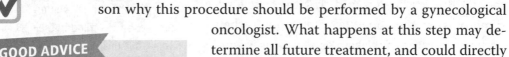

Ovarian cancer patients should be treated according to National Comprehensive Care Network guidelines. Unfortunately, though, a recent study of ovarian cancer patients in California found that only 35 percent of women were being treated according to these guidelines, and that those who were not missed out on a chance to add a year or more to their lives.

Treatments

SURGERY

The extent of surgery involved in treating epithelial ovarian cancer depends on its stage. Surgery generally involves a hysterectomy, a **bilateral salpingo-oophorectomy** (removal of both ovaries and both fallopian tubes), the removal of the **omentum** (the layer of fatty tissue that covers the contents of the abdomen), and removal of lymph nodes. Surgery for advanced ovarian cancer may require removal of other organs including part of the intestine, liver, and/or bladder to achieve "optimal" tumor debulking. In advanced ovarian cancer — a Stage IV cancer, characterized by liver and/or bone metastasis — chemotherapy prior to surgery may be performed in order to shrink the tumor.

Debulking refers to removing all signs of cancer larger then one centimeter. When performed successfully, this is known as complete or "optimal" debulking. If this is only done partially, it is called "sub-optimal debulking." Patients who are optimally debulked have a better prognosis. Doctors should be asked how often they operate on ovarian cancer patients and the percentage of cases in which they achieve optimal debulking.

Surgery for Germ Cell Ovarian Cancer

Ovarian cell tumors can be treated with a hysterectomy and bilateral salpingo-oophorectomy. If the cancer is in only one ovary, and the woman intends to bear children, only the one ovary containing the cancer and the fallopian tube may be removed, leaving the unaffected ovary, fallopian tube, and uterus in place.

Surgery for Ovarian Stromal Cancer

These cancers are usually confined to just one ovary, so if the tumor is localized, only that ovary may need removal. If the cancer has spread, surgery must be more extensive, and can range from a hysterectomy to a full debulking.

Surgery for Low Malignant-Potential Ovarian Tumor

This type of ovarian tumor can require the removal of the affected ovary, a hysterectomy, an even more involved surgery, or even debulking depending on how widespread the tumor cells are.

CHEMOTHERAPY

Along with surgery, aggressive chemotherapy is the basis of treatment for most types of ovarian cancer. A number of

DID YOU KNOW . . .

Ovarian cancer surgery is usually more extensive than most other types of cancer surgery due to the way the disease tends to spread. Like other cancers, ovarian cancer spreads from organ to organ. But unlike most other cancers, ovarian tumors also "shed," sending out cancerous seeds that can blanket the abdomen, for instance. This also raises the possibility of missing cancerous cells, which is why meticulous surgery is so necessary.

chemotherapy drugs are used in the treatment of ovarian cancer, and the types and number of rounds vary depending on the stage of the cancer.

"Chemotherapy can be administered traditionally, but in some cases, the method of administration can make a big difference, especially when it comes to **intraperitoneal (IP) therapy**," says Dr. Akers.

IP Chemotherapy

This is a treatment in which a catheter is placed in the abdomen to deliver chemotherapy directly into the pelvic area. A landmark study in 2006 found that this form of therapy extended survival by more than a year (15.9 months).

The National Cancer Institute took a rare step, one it reserves for major advances. It issued a "clinical announcement" to encourage doctors to use the IP treatment, and to urge patients to ask about it. Cancer specialists predicted that the announcement would lead to widespread changes in treatment, but as of this writing, experts say that is not the case.

"Giving chemotherapy this way gives the most concentrated dose of the drugs to the cancer cells in the abdominal cavity. The chemotherapy drugs are also absorbed into the bloodstream and so can reach cancer cells outside the abdominal cavity. The side effects are often more severe, though. But if you are a candidate for this type of chemotherapy it is important that you be offered it. This type of chemotherapy is also more likely to be offered at a cancer center of excellence," Dr. Akers notes.

HORMONE THERAPY

Hormones or hormone-blocking drugs are rarely employed to fight epithelial ovarian cancer, but they are more commonly used to treat stromal ovarian cancers. These drugs include **luteinizing-hormone-releasing hormone (LHRH) agonists**, which lower estrogen levels in premenopausal women, and **tamoxifen**, the anti-estrogen drug best known as a breast cancer fighter. **Aromatase inhibitors**, which lower estrogen levels in post-menopausal women, are also used for recurrences of stromal tumors.

TARGETED THERAPY

This newer type of cancer treatment uses drugs or other substances to identify and attack cancer cells while doing little damage to normal cells. **Avastin (bevacizumab)** is a targeted therapy that has been by far the most studied for ovarian cancer, although others are being researched as well.

RADIATION

Therapy of any type using radiation is rare in the treatment of ovarian cancer.

16

Soft Tissue Sarcoma

THERE IS A SAYING in medicine: If you hear hooves, look for horses, not zebras. This basically means that when a doctor evaluates symptoms, a common disease is more likely the one the patient will have. So, when Nancy Newsom Ridgway first showed her rheumatologist the swelling in her leg, he recommended that she put heat on it. "My doctor is very good, it's just that sarcomas are very rare," notes Ridgway, 63. When the swelling worsened, though, he referred her to an oncologist. "She scheduled me for surgery, but she assumed I had a lipoma," which is a benign fatty lump that grows beneath the skin.

The key reason why Nancy seeks to publicize her story is because her condition is, indeed, quite uncommon. "People need to have more awareness of this form of cancer, so they can get it checked out more quickly," added Nancy, whose tumor was surgically removed, and is now nearing the five-year survival mark. "I'm very hopeful, but I want everyone to know about this disease," she adds.

What Is Sarcoma?

The term "sarcoma" comes from the Greek word that means "fleshy growth." Soft tissue sarcomas occur in the body's connective tissue, including the muscles, blood vessels, nerves, tendons, cartilage, and fat. They can also occur in the **synovial tissue**, which is the tissue that cushions the joints.

"Most cancers come from organs and therefore are called carcinomas. Sarcomas come from the connective tissue in cells that occur all over the body. Any cell in the body that arises from the connective tissue, unfortunately, can be transformed into a sarcoma," says Dr. Gary Schwartz, associate director of the Herbert Irving Comprehensive Cancer Center and chief of hematology and oncology at Columbia University.

Statistics

About 12,000 adults are diagnosed with soft-tissue sarcoma each year, and 4,400 people succumb to the disease. About 50 percent of soft tissue sarcomas begin in the arm or leg, 40 percent in the torso or abdomen, and 10 percent in the head or neck. In addition there are many different sub-types of sarcoma, some arising from the muscle, others from the fat and other connective tissue cells. There are in fact over 50 different sarcoma sub-types, making this a very complicated tumor type as each of these sarcomas can act and behave differently. Therefore, the treatment plan chosen by your medical oncologist and sarcoma specialist is directly determined by the particular type of sarcoma you have.

People can develop a soft tissue sarcoma at any age, but they are more common in older adults, with 57 as the average age of diagnosis. Fifty-one is the average age that adults develop the most common type of bone sarcoma.

"Generally, it's not known why people develop sarcomas," says Dr. Schwartz, adding, "It really is a freak of nature. No one knows what happens to cause the genetic mutation that sets it off — it just happens."

There are a few rare genetic syndromes such as neurofibromatosis, Werner syndrome, or familial syndromes associated with p53 gene mutations — the mutation often found in those with soft tissue sarcoma.

Cancer survivors who received radiation for other cancers like breast cancer and lymphoma may develop sarcoma in that same region several years later. Occupational exposure to certain chemicals and other substances, including vinyl chloride, and phenoxyacetic acid (found in herbicides) and chlorophenols, which are used in wood preservative, can also increase risk.

Outcome and Survival Rates

More than 107,000 people in the United States today are living with sarcomas. Survival rates hinge on the grade of the disease, with a five-year survival rate for early stage, localized sarcomas at 83 to 90 percent. That drops to 54 percent for sarcomas that have spread to the lymph nodes. If a sarcoma spreads to distant parts of the body, the survival rate drops to 16 percent; however, if the sarcoma is located in an arm or leg, the five-year survival rates are slightly higher for each stage. Such sarcomas used to require amputation, but thanks to modern reconstruction techniques, this now only occurs in about five percent of cases.

GOOD ADVICE

Agent Orange, the herbicide used during the Vietnam War, is associated with an increased risk of sarcoma. If you are a Vietnam War veteran, you may be eligible for benefits. See the appendix for more information.

Types of Sarcoma

Instead of being classified according to cancer type, sarcomas are grouped according to the type of tissue from which the cancer developed. For instance, liposarcoma develops from fat tissue, while chondrosarcoma develops from cartilage cells.

SOFT TISSUE SARCOMA

While there are several types of soft tissue sarcomas, these are the most common:

Liposarcoma

This is the most common form of soft tissue tumor. Liposarcomas usually develop in the deep fatty tissue, and they occur most commonly in the thigh, behind the knee, the groin, the buttocks, or behind the abdominal cavity (retroperitoneum). Liposarcomas are usually malignant, and they most often occur in adults between 30 and 60 years of age. Men are slightly more likely to develop them.

Malignant Fibrous Histiocytoma (MFH)

These are the most common soft tissue sarcomas that occur in people between the ages of 50 and 70. They occur twice as often in men. There are four variations of MFH:

- Storiform-pleomorphic
- Myxoid malignant fibrous histiocytoma
- Malignant giant cell tumor of soft parts
- Inflammatory malignant fibrous histiocytoma

It is extremely important that the cancer be accurately diagnosed, because these sarcomas act quite differently. Storiform and myxoid MFH types are typically high-grade, fast-growing, aggressive tumors, while malignant giant cell MFH and inflammatory MFH types are slower growing and less likely to spread.

Stages of Soft Tissue Sarcoma

The stage of a soft tissue sarcoma is dependent on its grade, which denotes how fast-growing or aggressive it is.

STAGE I

Early soft tissue sarcomas are low-grade tumors of any type. Stage I tumors are slower growing, and they have not yet spread to the lymph nodes or to distant organs, such as the lungs or brain.

STAGE II

The tumor is larger than a Stage I tumor and graded higher, or more aggressive. Although the sarcoma has not yet spread to the lymph nodes, it is at high risk of doing so.

STAGE III

The tumor may or may not have spread to the lymph nodes, but it is a more aggressive grade than in Stage II. It has not yet spread to distant organs.

STAGE IV

The cancer can be any grade, but it has spread to the lymph nodes and/or to distant sites.

Signs and Symptoms

There are usually no symptoms in an early stage soft tissue sarcoma. As the sarcoma grows larger, it can cause these symptoms:

- A lump or swelling

- Pain

- A blockage in the stomach or gastrointestinal tract if the tumor is located in the abdomen

A lump or bump is usually the first symptom, and the time to get it seen is immediately, says Dr. Schwarz. "We all have lumps and bumps on our skin, but if you notice a new one, or one that changes, get to your internist and, if you aren't satisfied with the explanation or treatment, see a specialist. A delay in diagnosis clearly impacts curability," he adds.

Specific Diagnostic Tests

Imaging tests can be used to tentatively diagnose a sarcoma. These may include X-ray, CT scan, MRI, PET scan, and ultrasound. But the only way to confirm the diagnosis is with a biopsy.

The biopsy process may begin with a fine needle aspiration (FNA), in which a very small needle is placed into the tumor in order to extract tiny bit of tissue. If an examination of the cells finds the tumor may be a sarcoma, another type of biopsy will probably be done to remove a larger piece of tissue and confirm the diagnosis. This might be a core needle, incisional, or excisional biopsy. See chapter 2 for more information.

Treatments

Surgery, whenever possible, is the primary form of treatment for sarcomas, no matter what the stage. But the outcome of the surgery is dependent on the expertise of the surgeon, and while this is true for any cancer operation, it is particularly true of sarcoma, notes Dr. Schwartz. "You really do need to find a great surgeon. A lot of surgeons don't know how to handle a sarcoma tumor," he says.

This is true even of surgical oncologists because sarcomas are so rare, they may only have one or two opportunities to perform such a surgery throughout their careers. And sarcomas are more complex and difficult to deal with than many other types of cancers, which increases the risk when an operation is involved.

"When an inexperienced surgeon cuts into a tumor, there is a risk of cancer cells being spread around," says Dr. Schwartz. "These tumors can also wrap around blood vessels and nerves, so an experienced surgeon really needs to be the one who attempts to remove them.

"This is why, if you are diagnosed with a sarcoma or are suspected of having one, you need to find a doctor experienced in treating them, and these experts are at the top cancer centers," Dr. Schwartz advises.

In addition to surgery to remove the tumor, sarcomas located in the arms or legs may require delicate limb-sparing surgery, as well as reconstructive work later to avoid amputations that occurred commonly in the past.

In addition to surgery, radiation and chemotherapy can also be used, although chemotherapy plays a lesser role than does radiation, notes Dr. Schwartz.

TREATMENTS FOR THE STAGES OF SARCOMA
Stage I

If the tumor is small (less than five centimeters, or two inches across) and in the legs or arms, only surgery may be needed. Sometimes surgery is followed by radiation if the tumor is larger, or if the surgeon is unable to obtain clear margins, which means that there may still be cancer cells found close to the edges of the tissue that was removed. This is to prevent the cancer from recurring. For tumors occurring elsewhere in the body, like the head, neck, or abdomen, radiation and/or chemotherapy may be administered to shrink the tumor so that it can be surgically removed.

Stages II and III

Surgery alone is usually not considered enough to cure these larger sarcomas. If high-grade, these tumors tend to be more aggressive and capable of spreading to distant organs. If the tumor is removable, surgery is performed, followed by radiation and/or chemotherapy. If the tumor is not removable, patients may undergo radiation, chemotherapy, or a combination to shrink the tumor so it can be surgically removed. Except for rare circumstances, there is no proven benefit to undergoing chemotherapy after removing a sarcoma (so-called "adjuvant chemotherapy"), even for large and high-grade tumors.

Stage IV

Most sarcomas that have spread to distant sites are usually not curable, although a cure is possible if the main tumor and all of the areas where the tumor has spread (the metastases) can be surgically removed. But if this is impossible, surgery can be performed in very specific cases to remove as much of the main tumor and the metastases as possible.

RADIATION

Small sarcomas are generally treated with surgery alone, but the majority of these tumors are larger when diagnosed. In this case, both surgery and radiation are used. In combination with surgery, radiation therapy may reduce the chance of recurrence. Alternately, radiation may be used before surgery to shrink the tumor, thereby increasing the space between the tumor and vital organs, so the surgeon can better remove it. Radiation sterilizes cancer cells, damaging their DNA so they can't grow and spread.

PROTON THERAPY

Unlike conventional radiation, this therapy involves the use of a targeted proton beam, which destroys less healthy tissue, thus lowering the risk of both short-term and long-term side effects. Once viewed as controversial and expensive, it is becoming more accepted as treatment centers across our nation adopt it.

CHEMOTHERAPY

Chemotherapy is not as effective in treating most sarcomas as it is in other forms of cancer. Still, it can be used to treat symptoms and has been shown to improve survival in the metastatic setting. The most common types of chemotherapy drugs are **doxorubicin, ifosfamide, dacarbazine, gemcitabine,** and **docetaxel**. More recently the FDA approved an oral drug called **pazopanib** for patients who fail primary chemotherapy.

However, there are some kinds of sarcomas that are sensitive to chemotherapy, like **embryonal rhabdomyosarcoma (ERMS),** a fast-growing muscle malignancy, and synovial cell sarcoma. In such cases, chemotherapy may be used to shrink the tumor before surgery, and afterwards as well to kill any remaining cancer cells. As chemotherapy tends to be less effective for the treatment of many sarcomas, consideration should be given for participation in clinical trials where new agents are being evaluated to treat this host of diseases.

Recurrent Sarcoma

It is not uncommon for sarcoma to recur. A tumor can recur in the site of origin (locally), or it may appear in a distant site, like the lungs or the brain. If the sarcoma comes back locally, surgery may be performed again to remove it, or radiation can be administered if it was not performed before. Sarcoma often spreads to the lungs and when it does, it may be curable with surgery. If it has spread elsewhere, like to the brain, radiation is often used to relieve symptoms.

17

Testicular Cancer

WHEN MIKE CRAYCRAFT WAS diagnosed with testicular cancer, he was certain that he was going to die. Convinced that his time was short, the 33-year-old set about creating a bucket list. He even decided to throw a big going-away party for himself, but still kept his secret. "I had heard of testicular cancer, but I didn't know anything about a potential cure or odds of survival, so I just assumed I had a metastatic disease and I was going to die. I put off treatment for seven months."

Finally, Craycraft summoned the courage to face the disease head-on, and pursued a treatment plan. Seven years later, he is not only cancer-free, but he is also the founder of the Testicular Cancer Society, which he organized to help spread the word to other men.

What Is Testicular Cancer?

Part of the male reproductive system, the testicles (also referred to as the testes or gonads), are egg-shaped glands located in the scrotum, the pouch that hangs behind and below the penis. The testes' two main functions are to produce sperm and testosterone (the sex hormone responsible for male gender characteristics). Testicular cancer commonly occurs in only one testicle (but can also reside in both), and begins in the testicle itself.

The testes are composed of differing cells, all of which are capable of developing into one or more types of cancer. **Germ cells** are responsible for sperm production; **stromal cells** make up hormone-supportive tissue; **Leydig cells** are tasked with the production of androgens, such as testosterone; and **Sertoli cells'** role is to nourish germ cells. Typically, tumors developing from Leydig and Sertoli cells are benign.

Statistics

There are about 231,000 testicular cancer survivors in the United States today. The disease primarily occurs in young men between 15 and 35 years old; although rare, it is the most common form of cancer in this age group. Older men can develop testicular cancer as well, although this is less common. Testicular cancer occurs 4.5 times more often in Caucasian men than in African-Americans. The risk for other races falls somewhere in between.

It isn't known why men develop testicular cancer, but there are several factors that are linked with this disease. Although men with none of these risk factors can develop it, testicular cancer does occur more frequently in those who've had one or more testicles fail to descend after birth. The risk remains even if the testicle is surgically corrected.

Testicular cancer, while not known to be inherited, does seem to run in families, so having a father, brother, or uncle with the disease does slightly increase your risk. So do certain genetic conditions like Down syndrome and Klinefelter syndrome, a rare condition in which a male baby is born with an extra X (female) chromosome. Some studies show that men with HIV infection, particularly AIDS, are at higher risk of developing testicular cancer as well.

As stated, testicular cancer generally occurs only in one testicle, and rarely in the second testicle, but men with it are at increased risk of that occurring.

Outcome and Survival Rates

Of the approximately 8,600 men who will be diagnosed with testicular cancer this year, about 400 will lose their battle with it. Once considered incurable, testicular cancer is now one of the most curable of cancers. "This is a very gratifying cancer to treat because we do have good outcomes, even in advanced stages," says Dr. Elizabeth Henry, a Loyola University Medical School oncologist whose specialties include testicular cancer.

GOOD ADVICE

Men with fertility problems also are increased risk for testicular cancer and should be checked for it. This is also true for relatively young men who suffer a blood clot in their leg or a lung.

"Testicular cancer was difficult to treat until the mid-'70s, when we began to develop an understanding of it, and for the next 20 years, new chemotherapy protocols were developed to cure it," notes Dr. Henry.

The results have been impressive. For men with local disease, meaning the cancer has not spread beyond the testicles, the survival rate is 99 percent. For men with cancer that has spread to the **retroperitoneal lymph nodes** (lymph nodes in the back of the abdomen), the survival rate is about 96 percent, and for men with cancer that has spread to distant areas outside the testicles, like the lungs and the liver, the survival rate drops to 71 percent.

Types of Testicular Cancer

GERM CELL TUMORS

Testicular tumors that arise from the germ cells (which manufacture sperm) are known as GCTs. There are many different types, but they generally fall into two groups: seminomas and non-seminomas.

Seminoma

This form accounts for 40 percent of all testicular germ cell cancers. The cancer is usually just in the testes, but it can spread to the lymph nodes. For a cancer to be considered a seminoma, it must be pure seminoma. If any other cancer cells are found at all, it is labeled a "non-seminoma" testicular cancer.

Non-Seminoma

This is a common type of testicular cancer that tends to grow more quickly than seminoma. These tumors are often made up of more than one type of cell, and are identified according to their different cell types. Here are the following common types:

- Choriocarcinoma
- Embryonal carcinoma
- Teratoma
- Yolk sac tumor

Stages of Testicular Cancer

As with other forms of cancer, the stage at which it is found determines both its prognosis and treatment.

STAGE 0

Cancerous cells are found only in the testicle and tumor markers are not elevated.

STAGE I

The cancer is found only in the testicle. Tumor markers may be elevated.

STAGE II

The cancer is found in the testicle and the lymph nodes of the abdomen.

STAGE III

In addition to being found in the testicle and lymph nodes, the cancer has spread to distant parts of the body.

Metastatic Lung Cancer

Traveling via the lymph system, one of the most common areas to which testicular cancer spreads is the lungs. But a spread of testicular cancer to the lung does not carry with it the deadly connotation that being diagnosed with lung cancer does. "Testicular cancer is still testicular cancer, no matter where in the body it goes, and this means it is still highly curable with chemotherapy," Dr. Henry points out.

Signs and Symptoms

- A painless lump that occurs either on the sides or the front of the testicle
- An enlarged testicle or a swollen one
- Pain or discomfort, with or without a lump, in the testicle(s) or scrotum
- A change in the way the testicle feels
- A feeling of heaviness in the scrotum
- A dull ache in the abdomen or groin
- Breast tenderness or growth

"A mass, pain, or swelling in the testes is the most common presentation. Sometimes redness occurs. Some men are reluctant to bring such a problem to their doctor's attention, but if they notice anything unusual they really should," Dr. Henry says.

GOOD ADVICE

Testicular lumps are rare, so if you notice one, contact your doctor immediately. It may be a harmless lump but it must be checked in order to rule out testicular cancer.

Specific Diagnostic Tests

PHYSICAL EXAM

The doctor checks the testicles for any lumps or abnormalities. The doctor will also check the groin area, abdomen, armpits, and neck to check for any signs of lymph node swelling, and will also check the breasts for any swelling, enlargement, or tenderness.

BIOPSY

In most cases when cancer is suspected, the doctor orders a biopsy to confirm it. In the case of testicular cancer, though, this can be unwise. Since the testicles are located very close to the lymph nodes, taking a tissue sample to biopsy could result in spreading cancer cells. In addition, the procedure could also change the predictable route along which the cancer spreads — one of the reasons why this cancer is so comparatively easy to treat. **So if your doctor recommends a biopsy, get a second opinion.**

SCROTAL ULTRASOUND

This painless, non-invasive procedure employs sound waves used to produce images of inside the scrotum and testicles.

ORCHIECTOMY

If the ultrasound reveals a solid mass or other indication of testicular cancer, the surgeon will perform a procedure known as a **radical inguinal orchiectomy** to remove the entire testicle.

This is a surgical procedure in which an incision is made high up in the groin area and the entire testicle is removed. Then, the pathologist examines slices of tissue under a microscope to determine the type and the stage of the cancer. Since the entire testicle is removed, this can be curative for Stage I testicular cancer.

For appearance, some men to prefer to have prosthetic testicle implanted after surgery; however, this is optional. Since the implant serves no function, this is purely a matter of individual preference.

BLOOD TESTS AND TUMOR MARKERS

Testicular cancer tumors can secrete proteins or hormones into the bloodstream. These "tumor markers" can furnish important information as to the diagnosis, type of tumor, and the success of treatment. These tumor markers include: AFP (alpha-fetoprotein); beta-hCG (beta-human chorionic gonadotropin); and LDH (lactic acid dehydrogenase). Monitoring these markers enables your doctor to know if your diagnosis and tumor type are correct, and if you are responding to treatment.

OTHER IMAGING TESTS
Chest X-ray, CT (CAT), PET and **bone scans** may be used to see if the cancer has spread.

DID YOU KNOW . . .

Not all forms of testicular cancer produce tumor markers or elevated levels of these substances. You can have testicular cancer even if your tumor markers are normal. Also, these levels can appear elevated for reasons other than testicular cancer.

Treatments

As with other cancers, the treatment of testicular cancer depends on the stage as well as the aggressiveness of the tumor. "All men with testicular cancer will undergo surgery to have the affected testicle removed, and then the tumor is examined to determine the stage and how advanced it is," notes Dr. Henry.

One reason why testicular cancer is so treatable is because it spreads in a predictable pattern, unlike most other cancers. The two major modes of treatment are surgery and chemotherapy. "The more limited the disease, the more likely a surgical option will be offered. If the disease is more advanced, this makes it more likely that chemotherapy will be required," Dr. Henry explains. "Radiation can be used as well, although if this therapy is used at the beginning, it makes it less possible for it to be utilized later on."

The treatment for testicular cancer depends on whether the cancer is diagnosed while it is localized within the testicle or whether it has spread to the abdominal lymph nodes or to distant organs. It also depends on whether the tumor is a seminoma or non-seminoma.

GOOD ADVICE

A urologist is usually one of the first doctors consulted if a patient suspects he has testicular cancer, but once the diagnosis is confirmed, you should seek care from an expert experienced in treating testicular cancer. Such an expert is usually found at a large cancer center.

ORCHIECTOMY

This is the main treatment for testicular cancer, as noted. The following treatments listed are all in addition to this main treatment that calls for the removal of the affected testicle.

ACTIVE SURVEILLANCE

Also known also as "watchful waiting," active surveillance is for patients with early stage testicular cancer once the affected testicle has been removed and the tumor markers are normal, or they have returned to normal. This option involves close and active monitoring for recurrent cancer. It does avoid radiation and/or chemotherapy, but it involves blood tests, imaging tests, and frequent check-ups.

RADIATION

High-energy beams of radiation are used to destroy cancer cells left behind after the orchiectomy. A common schedule for testicular cancer calls for daily radiation treatments, five days a week for three to four weeks. See chapter 3 for more information.

CHEMOTHERAPY

Among treatments, chemotherapy has elicited by far the best response in testicular cancer sufferers, and is responsible for the turnaround in the survival rate for this disease. Chemotherapy is used more frequently for non-seminomas than seminoma tumors.

RETROPERITONEAL LYMPH NODE DISSECTION (RPLND)

This surgery is done if testicular cancer has spread and can produce a 50 percent to 75 percent cure rate — far higher than other types of metastatic cancer. This surgery removes the retroperitoneal lymph nodes that are located at the back of the abdomen. An incision is made down the middle of the abdomen to remove the lymph nodes. The removal of the lymph nodes is also known as a lymphadenectomy.

Recurrent Testicular Cancer

If testicular cancer returns after being treated, it may recur in the testicle, or in another part of the body. Recurrences tend to take place within the first two years of treatment, though they can happen as late as ten years after treatment. In this event, it's best to go to a top cancer center and see an expert who has experience in treating relapsed testicular cancer. Treatment for relapse depends on the type of treatment already performed. In some cases, a bone marrow transplant may be recommended to enable high doses of chemotherapy to be administered.

Preserving Fertility

The removal of a testicle does not affect a man's ability to achieve an erection or his ability to father children; however, treatment for testicular cancer can affect fertility. Therefore, if you are young, or think there is even a remote possibility you may want to father a child someday, you should discuss sperm banking with your doctor. Sperm banking involves providing sperm, which is frozen for later use. Ideally, sperm banking should take place before the removal of the testicle and the start of radiation and/or chemotherapy. Even men who have very low sperm counts (before cancer) should consider sperm banking.

"Many men will go on to recover their fertility, but we never know which ones, so we tell all patients it's a good idea for them to consider sperm banking," Dr. Henry says.

Men who did not store their sperm before treatment may still be able to father a child after treatment, depending on the amount and type of treatment used. But it's always best to make preparations beforehand, if possible.

Uterine Cancer

18

MARY LEONARD WAS 61 and past menopause when, one night after coming home from a meeting, she noticed she was bleeding. "My family history is riddled with cancer. My mother died of uterine cancer when I was young, and when my stepmother (though we didn't share a gene pool) began suffering repeated episodes of abnormal bleeding, she was diagnosed with uterine cancer as well, so I knew I should call my doctor immediately," recalls Leonard.

Leonard's gynecologist, who had treated both her mother and her stepmother, immediately ordered an ultrasound test and when, as expected, he found uterine cancer, he referred her immediately to a gynecologic oncologist. "It turned out to be uterine cancer, and the most aggressive form of it as well," says Leonard. Her lymph nodes all tested negative, though; the disease hadn't spread, and her prognosis was good.

"I tell everyone that if you experience a symptom and your gut tells you something is wrong, act immediately. My chance of survival would have been far less if I had waited," she says.

What Is Uterine Cancer?

Also known as endometrial cancer, uterine cancer is the most common gynecological cancer. It occurs in the uterus — the hollow, pear-shaped organ designed to nourish an unborn baby. The uterus is part of a woman's reproductive system and is located between the bladder and the rectum. There are many uterine tumors that are benign, but malignant tumors are cancerous and are dangerous because they can spread to other parts of the body.

The vast majority (95 percent) of uterine cancers are known as **endometrial carcinomas**, because they arise from the endometrial lining of the uterus. A tiny minority (five percent) are sarcomas that arise from the muscle cells. This chapter covers endometrial cancers. Sarcoma cancers that arise in the uterus are treated as sarcomas and are covered in chapter 16.

Statistics

There are approximately 250,000 women who are uterine cancer survivors in the United States. About 50,000 women are diagnosed with uterine cancer each year, making it the fourth most common cancer. It is estimated that 8,200 women will die from the disease, which makes uterine cancer the eighth most common cause of cancer death for women in the United States.

While any woman can develop uterine cancer, certain risk factors increase the probability. The main risk factor is age. Uterine cancer usually occurs in women who are over 60 and past menopause.

Overweight women are more at risk for uterine cancer because fat produces estrogen, the female sex hormone, which is believed to be a contributor to this form of cancer. Eating a high-fat diet is linked to increased risk as well.

Also, while uterine cancer is not directly inherited, it is estimated that one in 10 cases are due to an inherited predisposition to the disease. This includes women with the following characteristics:

DID YOU KNOW . . .

The longer a woman's body is exposed to estrogen, the higher her risk of uterine cancer. This includes women who began menstruating at an early age, those who have never been pregnant, and women who have late menopause.

- Women who developed uterine cancer at a younger-than-expected age (less than five percent of cases are diagnosed in women under 40)

- Those with relatives who developed the disease

- Women with a history of colon polyps before the age of 40

- Women who inherited HNPCC (see chapter 8),which is primarily associated with an increased colon and endometrial cancer risk

- Women with endometrial hyperplasia, which is an overgrowth of cells in the uterine lining

- Diabetics

- Breast, colon, and ovarian cancer survivors

- Cancer survivors who have taken the breast cancer drug tamoxifen (Nolvadex) or who underwent radiation in the pelvic area for other cancers

- Women who used estrogen alone as a form of hormone replacement therapy

DID YOU KNOW . . .

Women commonly develop growths in the uterus that are not cancerous. These include fibroids (benign tumors that develop in the uterine muscle); endometriosis (the growth of endometrial tissue on the outside of the uterus); or an endometrial polyp.

Outcome and Survival Rates

Uterine cancer is among the more curable forms of cancer. The five-year survival rate for a woman with a local uterine cancer at diagnosis is now about 97 percent. If the cancer has spread outside the uterus, but only to the cervix, the rate drops to 69 percent, and then to roughly 60 percent when it spreads to the pelvic area. The five-year survival rate drops to 16 percent if the cancer has spread to the lymph nodes where it can reach more distant organs. However, most uterine cancers are diagnosed well before then.

Types of Uterine Cancer

Adenocarcinoma is the most common form of endometrial cancer. These tumors arise from the glands of the endometrium. They are also referred to as **endometrioid adenocarcinoma**. As the name denotes, these tumors are made up completely of endometrial cells. There are other, rarer forms of endometrial cancer that are made up of other types of cells or a mixture of cells, but endometrioid adenocarcinomas make up 80 percent of endometrial cancer.

Stages of Uterine (Endometrial) Cancer

As with other forms of cancer, the stage at which it is found predicates its treatment and also its prognosis. These are the stages of endometrial cancer; it is important to remember, though, that there are survivors at every stage of the disease, no matter when it was diagnosed. Also, like other cancers, uterine cancer is categorized according to grade, which is a rating that denotes how slow-growing or aggressive the cancer is believed to be; the higher the grade, the more aggressive the cancer.

GOOD ADVICE

Although uterine cancer is highly curable, it is still a potentially dangerous form of cancer so proper diagnosis, staging, and treatment are necessary right from the start. The gynecologic oncologis, who specializes in the treatment of cancers of the female reproductive system, is the doctor who has the most training and experience in treating this disease.

STAGE I

The cancer is found in the uterus only. The survival rate for this earlier stage of cancer is 90 percent.

STAGE II

Endometrial cancer cells are found in the connective tissue of the cervix (the narrow opening that connects the uterus to the vagina), but the cancer has not spread outside that organ.

STAGE III

The cancer has spread throughout the uterus and the cervix, and may also have spread to other organs in the reproductive system, including the fallopian tubes, the ovaries, and the vagina, but it has not spread outside the pelvic region.

STAGE IV

The cancer has spread beyond the pelvis to the abdomen and the lymph nodes in the groin, from which it can spread to distant parts of the body as well.

"The outcome for cancers that are caught in the early stage and are of low-grade (meaning non-aggressive) has been fairly excellent all along. But we are also doing better with the more aggressive cancers that are more likely to recur," says Dr. Peter Frederick, gynecologic oncologist and the director of minimally invasive surgery for such cancers at Roswell Park Cancer Institute in Buffalo, New York.

About 70 percent of such recurrences happen within three years of the initial treatment. Symptoms may be similar to the initial appearance of uterine cancer.

One of the most important factors in the treatment of endometrial cancer is accurate staging of the tumor. But this is not easy, because imaging tests done prior to surgery do not give complete information, and the only way to definitively stage the tumor is after surgery, says Dr. Frederick. "For those cases where staging of cancer is appropriate, it's very important to accurately stage a uterine cancer, because if the patient undergoes inappropriate or incomplete surgery, she may be undertreated and need a second operation, or overtreated and subjected to unnecessary radiation."

Signs and Symptoms

- Abnormal bleeding after menopause
- Pain during sexual intercourse
- Difficult or painful urination
- Pain in the pelvis

An abnormal, blood-streaked discharge from the vagina is the most common symptom of uterine cancer.

Specific Diagnostic Tests

The following section describes the tests that are specifically performed to diagnose uterine cancer. They may be done in addition to general cancer diagnostic testing. See chapter 2 for more information.

PELVIC EXAMINATION

The doctor feels the uterus, vagina, ovaries, fallopian tubes, bladder, and rectum to check for any unusual changes. A Pap test may also be done. This test is not done to diagnose uterine cancer, but may find abnormal glandular cells caused by it.

GOOD ADVICE

While most uterine cancer occurs after menopause, Dr. Frederick notes that diagnoses in younger women are becoming more common, perhaps related to the increasing incidence of obesity. Any post-menopausal woman who experiences bleeding or a bloody vaginal discharge should see her doctor as soon as possible.

TRANSVAGINAL ULTRASOUND

This test utilizes a wand-like instrument placed in the vagina that emits sound waves to produce an image of the organs of the reproductive system.

OTHER IMAGING TESTS

X-ray, CT scans, PET scans, and MRI scans may be used to show any tumors or abnormalities.

ENDOMETRIAL BIOPSY

The doctor inserts a small tube into the uterus through the cervix and, using suction, removes a small sample of tissue that is then studied under the microscope.

HYSTEROSCOPY

The doctor uses a thin, lighted tube, called a hysteroscope, to examine the inside of the uterus.

D&C

Formally known as "dilation and curettage," this procedure, like a biopsy, also removes cellular tissue for examination. It is often performed in combination with a hysteroscopy, allowing the doctor to view the lining of the uterus during the procedure. Once uterine tissue has been removed either during a biopsy or D&C, the sample is checked for cancer cells.

LYMPHADENECTOMY

This surgery to remove the lymph nodes is done to definitively determine the exact stage and aggressiveness of the uterine cancer. It is done if cancer cells were found in the lymph nodes or at the same time as a hysterectomy.

The necessity of this procedure is controversial. Some doctors recommend it be done for all cases of uterine cancer, including the apparently localized, earlier stages to help determine the need for additional therapy after surgery, while others reserve it for patients with more advanced disease. In any case, this is major surgery that carries with it the risk of side effects, so whether to undergo this procedure is an important decision. Again, those diagnosed with uterine cancer should be treated by a gynecologic oncologist, who will best determine the need for this procedure.

Treatments

The protocol for addressing uterine cancer depends on whether the cancer is caught while in an early stage, or at a later state when it has spread beyond the uterus. In most cases, uterine cancer is initially treated with surgery, and the type depends on the stage of the cancer. Radiation, chemotherapy, hormone therapy, or a combination of these may be used as a course of treatment.

SURGERY

This is the initial treatment for uterine cancer. Depending on the stage of the cancer, the surgeon will perform either a simple hysterectomy (removal of the uterus and cervix), or a radical hysterectomy (removal of the uterus, cervix, the upper part of the vagina and the surrounding area). A bilateral salpingo-oophorectomy (removal of both fallopian tubes and ovaries) as well as the removal of lymph nodes is also usually performed.

"The cornerstone of treatment for uterine cancer is a hysterectomy, with removal of the uterus and cervix, both ovaries, and the fallopian tubes," says Dr. Frederick. Chemotherapy and/or radiation are also used to treat local uterine cancers that are more aggressive, or those that have spread. "Radiation or hormone therapy may be preferable to surgery for women who are elderly or frail," he adds.

Minimally to moderately invasive techniques include laparoscopic surgery, being performed through several very small incisions, with abdominal surgery requiring an incision measuring about five inches.

RADIATION

High-energy radiation kills cancer cells by damaging their ability to multiply. There are two types of radiation that can be used to treat uterine cancer. **External-beam radiation** therapy delivers treatment from a machine outside the body. **Brachytherapy** delivers treatments by using radioactive sources that are placed into the vagina, uterus and/or surrounding tissues to kill the cancer cells. See chapter 3 for more information on radiation.

CHEMOTHERAPY

As with many other forms of cancer, chemotherapy can be used to treat uterine cancer after surgery to make sure that all the cancer cells have been eradicated or in more advanced stages of cancer as well. Chemotherapy can also render a woman infertile or induce early menopause. See chapter 3 for more information.

HORMONE THERAPY

This method is used to slow the growth of uterine cancer cells. Hormone therapy for uterine cancer involves the sex hormone progesterone, administered in pill form. Hormone therapy may be used for women who cannot have surgery or radiation therapy, or in combination with other types of treatment. Side effects of hormone therapy include fluid retention, increase in appetite, and weight gain. Women in their childbearing years may have changes in their menstrual cycle.

Post-Diagnosis

The Psychological Impact of Cancer

THERE ARE MANY TYPES of life-threatening illnesses that people deal with all the time, and after they recover, their lives go on much as before. This is not true of cancer. Cancer changes you, not only physically, but emotionally as well.

"I don't think anybody can go through cancer and not have a change in perspective," says Ginny Dixon. She was a young journalist working at the *Los Angeles Times* when she was stricken with ovarian cancer 21 years ago. "Back then, I thought about winning Pulitzer Prizes, but after my diagnosis, that didn't matter in the same way that it did before. Cancer gives you a sense of urgency. You think you have forever and, all of a sudden, you don't," Dixon recalls.

"I think, universally, that every person who's just been diagnosed comes to the stark realization that they are dealing with a potentially life-threatening illness. And even though they are told, 'this is a small cancer, it's in an early stage, and likely curable,' most everyone knows someone who was told those very same words, and then they died of cancer. So being told you have cancer is a terrifying experience," says Dr. Mary Jane Massie, a board-certified psychiatrist at Memorial Sloan Kettering Cancer Center.

Not everyone reacts to cancer the same way, of course, but it's important to recognize that most patients and their families face some degree of depression, anxiety, and fear over a cancer diagnosis. But you don't have to tough it out alone.

Many hospitals and cancer centers already have procedures in place to routinely screen cancer patients for emotional distress and either treat them or refer them for help, and their number is growing. Beginning in 2015, the Commission on Cancer, which accredits centers that treat about 70 percent of all new cancers diagnosed in the United States, will require providers to perform such an evaluation and refer patients to programs for help.

The following are emotional types of distress that cancer patients often experience. For information on where to get help now, see the appendix.

Stress

Stress is the body's response to the perception of threat. This response dates back to prehistory, when man was faced with such perils as the sight of an approaching saber-tooth tiger. The body unleashes hormones, like adrenaline, that increase heart rate and blood flow to the legs, and heighten alertness and reaction time. Known as the "fight or flight" response, we are hard-wired to experience it. When the threat recedes, the body relaxes and hormone levels decline.

At least, that's how it works with short-term stress, or shock, such as learning you've been fired. But one of the reasons cancer is so emotionally taxing is because you have to deal with the initial shock of the diagnosis, and then with long-term stress as you face daily life with the disease. Thus, cancer produces both short-term and chronic stress.

Chronic stress means that, instead of subsiding, these hormones remain in your system and can damage your body, including your immune system. So, while there is no scientific evidence that stress actually causes cancer, it's been demonstrated that long-term stress has harmful biological effects, including impairing immune function, thus diminishing your body's ability to fight cancer.

Long-term stress also impacts your ability to effectively handle life's daily demands and can result in unhealthy eating habits, alcohol or drug abuse, inactivity, or social isolation — all factors that can negatively impact your cancer prognosis.

Symptoms of Long-Term Stress:

- Becoming easily agitated, frustrated, and moody
- Feeling overwhelmed
- Having difficulty relaxing and quieting your mind
- Feeling bad about yourself (low self-esteem)
- Feeling lonely and isolated
- Irritability
- Avoiding others

Depression

Sadness and grief are normal emotions when you are dealing with cancer. But these are emotions that are transient. Depression is more than sadness; it is a deeper sense of despair that doesn't go away by itself. In cancer patients, depression can be dangerous, because it not only diminishes your quality of life, but may also impair your ability to go about taking steps that could help ensure your survival.

Depression not only robs one of enjoyment of life, it also can pose a true threat to cancer survival. An analysis of 26 studies looked at a total of 9,417 cancer patients and found that those with depressive symptoms had a 25 percent higher risk of dying, and that this number rose to 39 percent in those diagnosed with either major or minor depression.

Cancer patients with depression report high pain scores, have a harder time making decisions about their treatment, and lack the ability to follow through on their treatment plans. Depression can negatively affect their ability to communicate with their loved ones as well.

Symptoms of Clinical Depression:

- Ongoing sad, hopeless or "empty mood" for most of the day

- Loss of interest or pleasure in almost all activities most of the time
- Major weight loss (not due to dieting) or weight gain
- Feeling slowed down or restless and agitated almost every day, enough for others to notice
- Extreme tiredness (fatigue) or loss of energy
- Trouble sleeping with early waking, sleeping too much, or not being able to sleep
- Trouble focusing thoughts, remembering, or making decisions
- Feeling guilty, worthless, or helpless
- Frequent thoughts of death or suicide (not just fear of death), or suicide plans or attempts

If five or more of these symptoms occur nearly every day for two weeks or more, or are severe enough to interfere with your normal activities, make an appointment with a mental health professional, the American Cancer Society recommends. Also, if you are having serious thoughts of suicide and/or have thought out a plan, get immediate help by calling the **National Suicide Prevention Lifeline** at **(800) 273-8255**.

GOOD ADVICE

Creating a blog or journaling about the cancer experience may lessen depression. A UCLA study of breast cancer patients found the women who did so reported less depression, better mood, and an enhanced appreciation for life. One way to create a personal blog is available on CaringBridge.org, an organization discussed a bit later in this chapter.

Anxiety

Along with depression, anxiety is a very common emotional response that cancer patients experience at different times during their treatment, which may persist for a long time afterwards as well.

Anxiety is a feeling of fear, unease, and worry. Generalized anxiety can be due to many reasons. Most of those who've experienced it cannot pin down a source for their anxiety, but when it comes to cancer patients, there's usually no need to cast about for the cause. A cancer diagnosis often brings with it anxiety, which can manifest anytime throughout the course of the disease, including during the initial diagnosis phase, treatment, or later on, when treatments have concluded and the individual is in recovery.

Sometimes anxiety permeates a cancer patient's day, but they can also experience sudden and acute "panic attacks." These stormy periods of anxiety occur suddenly and without warning, often reaching their worst within 10 minutes, and then begin to subside. Their symptoms can be so severe that the person believes they are having a heart attack.

Symptoms of Anxiety:

- Anxious facial expression
- Uncontrolled worry
- Trouble solving problems and focusing thoughts
- Muscle tension (the person may look tense or tight)
- Trembling or shaking
- Restlessness, feeling keyed-up or on-edge
- Dry mouth
- Irritability or angry outbursts (grouchy or short-tempered)
- Shortness of breath
- Chest tightness

If you are experiencing anxiety symptoms most of the day, nearly every day, and they are interfering with your life, consider contacting a mental health professional, the American Cancer Society says.

Joy and Cancer

You may be wondering what a section on joy is doing in a book about cancer. Well, it is impossible to conclude a discussion about the psychological effects of cancer without mentioning the fact that some cancer survivors interviewed for this book said that they have found a profound sense of joy in their experience. Chief among them is Joy Huber (ironically), whose experience with faith is related later in this chapter.

In her book, *Cancer with Joy*, Huber relates stories from 10 cancer survivors bent on finding hope, happiness, and, yes, joy from their experiences. (Actually 11 — Joy always likes to throw in a bonus.) They are stories of people of all ages, with different types of cancer, all from different walks of life. But what their stories have in common is their learned appreciation of the small things in life, their sense of gratitude, and their sense of humor

— all of which helped keep their spirits and the spirits of those around them aloft.

The stories in Joy's book underscore the fact that not everyone feels the same emotions when dealing with cancer. Also, it's not uncommon for emotions to seesaw. Everyone is unique, so honor your own feelings and emotions during this highly-charged, challenging time.

Dealing with Family and Friends

Only you can decide how and when you want to tell someone that you have cancer. Obviously, your spouse or partner very well may have been with you throughout the diagnostic process, but there are other family members or friends you will need to tell, and your employer as well.

In these days of instant social media, it's very valuable to realize that you have the power to tell who you want, and to do it in your own time. When Brett Johnson was diagnosed with brain cancer, for instance, he took some time to decide who he wanted to tell, and then went about it in an organized fashion.

Like many adults facing cancer, he found it most difficult to tell his parents.

"My mother was 79 at the time I was diagnosed with a brain tumor. She's very mentally vibrant and she's physically in good shape, but it I felt awful having to tell her. She had been dealing with my father's health, and I had gradually assumed the role of comforting her, so this was a huge shock for her," says Johnson. Once he did tell his mother, though, he found that she was able to handle the news. Not only that, but in 2013, Johnson's mother accompanied him and his brother on the "Boston Brain Tumor Walk," an event for which Johnson's mother trained.

But Brett also had to inform his voice students, as well as the people who hired him to perform. "I realized we had a huge number of people to tell so I decided to be honest with my network right up front," he says. But, as he faced brain surgery, he also knew the constant stream of inquiries from friends would soon be overwhelming. But a resource that he and many other survivors interviewed for this book found very helpful is a site run by a non-profit organization called CaringBridge.

CaringBridge.org provides easy-to-use tools so you can set up a protected website on which you can share as much — or as little — information as you please. You provide friends and family with the link through which they can access updates. Blogs are not only written by cancer patients, but can be created for any other type of serious disease. See the appendix for more information.

Telling close family members that you have cancer is hard, but this task is even more difficult when you are the parent of young children. Children are very sensitive and tend to pick up on far more cues and information than they're given credit for, and when they are not confronted with honest, accurate (and of course age-appropriate) information, they tend to suspect the worst. Talking to your patient advocate or social worker can help you decide what and how to tell them.

Young children (up to eight years old) will not need a lot of detailed information, while older children (eight to 12 years) and teens will need to know more. Teens, who are testing their independence and limits, will have very different concerns from the five-year-old child of a cancer patient, the American Cancer Society notes.

The organization also emphasizes that all children need to know the following as a minimum:

- The name of the cancer
- The part of the body that is affected
- How it will be treated
- How their own lives will be affected

Some hospitals and cancer centers also have support groups for children whose parents are dealing with cancer. The Children's Treehouse Foundation has a listing of cancer support groups for children and Kids Konnected is an organization that creates such groups. (See appendix.)

DID YOU KNOW . . .

We live in an age of intense social media, where it sometimes seems that everyone we know has access to all the details of our lives, especially through postings on Facebook. To eliminate over-sharing, some people prefer to get off Facebook, but you can also adjust your settings so people can't post on your page, or you can restrict certain people from seeing your updates.

The Role of Faith

Does prayer heal us? Although the role that faith plays in medicine may be controversial, it impossible to underestimate the role that faith has played in the lives of the many cancer survivors who shared their stories in this book.

Joy Huber, for instance, considers her faith to be one of her greatest tools in helping her deal with advanced non-Hodgkin's lymphoma. "After I was diagnosed with cancer, I kept praying the Lord's Prayer. One phrase kept coming back to me: 'Thy will be done on earth as it is in Heaven.' As I prayed, I was reminded that God has a plan and purpose for all of our lives. So I decided that I was just going to say, 'Thy will be done,' and I made that my mantra. And I found that asking God to walk me through this journey strengthened me," she recalls.

When people talk about the power of faith, they are generally referring to two types of prayer: intercessory prayer, which involves having someone pray for someone else at a distance, and the personal act of praying. While studies show the power of intercessory prayer to be mixed, the personal act of praying can confer many benefits, including the reduction of stress, notes Herbert Benson, MD, the cardiologist and Harvard professor whose bestseller *The Relaxation Response* helped to bring validation to the mind-body connection. Using Buddhist meditation, he demonstrated how this type of practice can play a significant role in reducing stress.

In addition, researchers have found that people who pray regularly are less likely to suffer from depression and anxiety, report more satisfaction in life, and report lesser amounts of pain. If you are not religious, some of the benefits of prayer, in terms of relaxation, can also be achieved through meditation.

Support Groups

Over the past 40 years, a vast network of support groups has emerged for people who are dealing with cancer. This form of support stemmed from the late 1970s and received a boost when a study in 1989 reported that breast cancer patients who participated in a support group coped better and lived longer. This resulted in a demand for support groups, and today there is a wide variety of support groups available. You can choose from groups that you attend in person, those that are run in chat rooms or on the Internet, and those that are telephone supported.

There are many different ways to find support groups. There are groups that are run by cancer organizations that cover virtually every type of cancer. There are also support groups that are run by cancer treatment centers and through hospitals, as well as groups that are formed by cancer survivors and advocates.

In addition, there are different types of organizations. Some offer education, some offer opportunities for recreation and socializing, and others are formed for caregivers. Still other groups are involved with advocacy, raising awareness, and fundraising for cancer-related causes.

The scientific evidence on whether support groups are beneficial is mixed, so whether or not to join one really comes down to your own personal decision. Some people report that they find tremendous emotional help in such groups; others are less enthusiastic. The choice is yours. If you think you might, though, it could be very worthwhile for you to check out the possibility, and, if you don't feel comfortable with the one you try, explore another. Check the appendix for more information.

Find a Mentor . . . or Become One

Having a mentor to help you through the cancer treatment process is another excellent way of finding support. When Joy Huber was diagnosed at 33, she was faced with not just becoming a cancer patient, but a young adult one, at that. "When you are diagnosed with cancer, you desperately want to find someone who will understand. I tried to talk to my friends, but I found that their only experience with cancer was through an older relative, so they had no idea what I felt like," she recalls.

Huber found Imerman's Angels, an organization that matches cancer patients with survivors, to be invaluable. Known as "Mentor Angels," the organization matches cancer survivors with patients according to age, gender, and type of cancer. "A Mentor Angel is walking, talking, living proof and inspiration that cancer can be beaten," the organization notes.

Several of the cancer survivors interviewed for this book mentioned Imerman's Angels, but there are other mentoring organizations as well, which can be found in the appendix. Many cancer survivors also find volunteering for such an organization helps them immeasurably. So, whether you get a mentor or eventually become one yourself (or both), mentoring can be an excellent choice for easing the emotional burden of cancer survival.

Cancer Survivor Issues

20

ANTONIO DIVINE AWOKE ONE morning to discover the lower part of his body was completely immobile. He spent weeks in the hospital undergoing tests for such serious diseases as amyotrophic lateral sclerosis (ALS, also known as Lou Gehrig's disease) and multiple sclerosis, all of which came back negative.

Gradually Divine's condition improved, although the cause of his ailment remained a mystery. Finally, a neurologist came up with the answer. The cause of Divine's problem was the chemotherapy he was given 18 years before, when, at 26, had undergone a very aggressive course to rid his lungs of cancer. "Back then, no one mentioned anything about what would happen after my cancer treatment," Divine recalls.

This is changing. The good news is that more cancer patients are alive now than ever before. Recent figures show an estimated 13.7 million people are living with a history of cancer — a figure that is expected to jump to almost 18 million by 2022.

Just because treatment ends doesn't mean that the challenge of cancer is over. There are many issues that cancer survivors face, which are only now being recognized. A positive note, though, is that with this awareness comes a great increase in the number of resources that are available to deal with them.

Who Is a Cancer Survivor?

The American Cancer Society defines a cancer survivor as a person falling into one of three distinct phases: the time of diagnosis to the end of initial treatment; the transition from treatment to extended survival; and long-term survival. This chapter focuses on long-term survival and covers medical, emotional, and lifestyle issues that can make the difference between not only in surviving cancer, but living healthy for the rest of your life.

Why Cancer Survivorship Plans Are Important

One of the profound changes in the field of cancer treatment is the focus on medical issues that cancer survivors face. This much-needed trend began about a decade ago and is now becoming a requirement for cancer treatment center accreditation.

Such survivorship plans can help doctors diagnose potential cancer recurrences and secondary cancers earlier. But they also are designed to screen cancer patients for other serious diseases and encourage them to institute and maintain healthy lifestyle changes. In addition, research shows they help cancer survivors feel empowered.

The need for such plans arose with the realization that, although cancer patients are likely to be monitored while they are under their doctor's care, this scrutiny ends once treatment does, and so there is no follow-through with care years later.

"It can be difficult for patients after their treatment ends. It's been found that a lot of cancer survivors do not get the care they need so their treatment tends to slip through the cracks," says Dr. Christine Hill-Kayser, a physician at the University of Pennsylvania Medical Center.

According to the Institute of Medicine, such survivorship plans should include information on the following:

- Late effects of cancer treatments; their symptoms and treatment

- Recommendations for medical screening
- Psychological effects
- Genetic counseling recommendations
- Recommendations for a healthy lifestyle
- Effective cancer prevention options
- Financial issues
- Referrals for follow-up care
- A list of support resources

The Three Factors of Cancer Survivorship

Living well after cancer depends on these important factors:

- Recognizing the late effects of cancer treatment
- Recognizing the psychological impact of cancer treatment
- Living a healthy lifestyle

Cancer Treatment's "Late Effects"

It's well-recognized that cancer treatments — including surgery, radiation, and medications like chemotherapy, hormonal treatment, and even the new targeted cancer drugs — although life-saving, also carry detrimental effects. Problems that occur during treatment (side effects) and persist are known as **long-term effects**. Diseases or conditions that may occur months, or even years after cancer treatment has ended are referred to as **late effects**.

In this section, you'll learn all about the potential late effects of cancer treatment. It's important to remember, though, that many people who have been treated for cancer do not experience these late effects. But knowing about them and discussing them with your healthcare provider is essential for living well after cancer.

CARDIAC ISSUES

Heart problems due to cancer treatment occur so commonly that there is now a new medical field called **cardioncology,** which focuses on heart damage/disease due to oncological treatment.

One chief cause of damage to the heart is radiation treatment. Radiation exposure causes the heart's coronary arteries (the vessels that bring blood to the heart) to thicken, which in turn causes

atherosclerosis — the disease process that results in coronary heart damage, which can lead to heart attack. This is particularly a danger when radiation it is administered to the chest area, as is done in the treatment of breast and lung, and non-Hodgkin's lymphoma.

Chemotherapy and radiation can also put excessive strain on the heart muscle, which can cause congestive heart failure, a condition that weakens the heart so that it can no longer pump blood efficiently. These treatments can also damage one or more of the heart's four valves, as well as the **pericardium** — the sac that surrounds the heart. In addition, these cancer treatments can cause high blood pressure, high cholesterol, and the tendency to gain weight, all of which contribute to heart problems.

Chemotherapy, especially the class of drugs called anthracyclines, was once considered a culprit in causing cardiac problems, but now the new, targeted cancer therapies, which are generally considered less toxic overall, are being found to cause heart damage as well. These include **Herceptin (trastuzumab)**, the HER2-targeted antibody used in breast cancer, as well the tyrosine inhibitors **Gleevec (imatinib)** and **Sutent (sunitinib)**.

DID YOU KNOW . . .

Herceptin is one of the major advances in breast cancer, but this drug is now implicated in the development of heart failure, so it is recommended that baseline tests be performed to evaluate the heart's pumping ability before treatment begins.

DIABETES

Diabetes is a metabolic disease in which the body doesn't produce or properly use insulin, the hormone that converts sugar and starch into energy. Some studies have found that steroid and some chemotherapy drugs can cause diabetes, so cancer survivors should have their blood glucose levels monitored.

REDUCED FERTILITY OR INFERTILITY

Cancer treatment can impact both men and women, either reducing or preventing their ability to conceive children.

For men, temporary or permanent infertility can occur when treatment affects the endocrine system, which includes the glands or other organs necessary to make hormones and sperm. Reduced fertility or infertility can occur with surgical treatments for prostate or testicular cancer, as well as with radical surgery for bladder and colon cancer. It can also be caused by chemotherapy, hormonal, and other drug treatments for different types of cancer. There are ways to preserve fertility, including sperm banking, but these need to be addressed before cancer treatment begins.

Many types of cancer treatment can temporarily or permanently affect a woman's ability to bear children. These include surgical removal of organs involved in the women's reproductive cycle or the pelvic lymph glands, the use of chemotherapy and other types of cancer drugs, and radiation of the whole body, the reproductive area, or the pituitary gland in the brain. Cancer treatment can also cause premature menopause in women, which not only affects their ability to bear children, but such hormonal changes can also cause osteoporosis, the bone thinning disease.

There are many ways to preserve a woman's ability to bear children, but again, these must be discussed before cancer treatment begins. However, a study reported in the *Journal of Clinical Oncology* found that, although most younger women are concerned about their ability to bear children, nearly one-third did not recall discussing this topic with their doctor and only a small number had decided to take advantage of methods to preserve their fertility. No matter what your gender, talk to your doctor before undergoing treatment if you think you might one day wish to have children.

SECONDARY CANCER

No one who has gone through cancer treatment wants to consider that they may develop a secondary cancer, but unfortunately, cancer survivorship comes with this inherent risk. Sometimes such a cancer may occur naturally, just as the first cancer did. But treatment with radiation, chemotherapy, or other drug agents may predispose a person to develop a secondary cancer as well, even years later.

Radiation can shrink cancers, but can also cause them. Radiation can cause leukemia or solid tumors (these usually occur at least 10 to 15 years after treatment ends) and the risk increases with the administered dosage. Risk also appears greater in people who were younger when treated.

Chemotherapy has also been linked to the development of leukemia, and some types of drugs are more likely to cause this blood cancer than are others.

PERIPHERAL NEUROPATHY

Many chemotherapy drugs can cause nerve damage, resulting in a condition known as **chemotherapy-induced peripheral neuropathy**. Peripheral neuropathy is a well-known side effect of some chemotherapy drugs that damage the nerves that control sensations and movements in the arms and legs, as well as the bladder and bowel.

Often, this form of peripheral neuropathy occurs during cancer treatment, but it can also persist afterwards or even become apparent later on. Surgery and/or radiation also can sometimes cause peripheral neuropathy. These are some of the major symptoms of peripheral neuropathy:

- Pain (may be there all the time or come and go in the form of shooting or stabbing pain)
- Burning
- Tingling ("pins and needles" feeling or electric, shock-like pain)
- Loss of feeling (can be numbness or just less ability to sense pressure, touch, heat, or cold)
- Trouble using your fingers to pick up or hold things; dropping things
- Balance problems
    - Trouble with tripping or stumbling while walking
    - Muscle weakness

Peripheral neuropathy can also cause blood pressure changes, trouble swallowing, difficulty passing urine, and decreased or no reflexes. If you notice symptoms of peripheral neuropathy, notify your healthcare provider and, if this occurs post-treatment, make sure they are aware of your medical history.

Specific Late Effects Based on Cancer Type

Here is a breakdown of specific medical conditions that survivors of the following types of cancers are at increased risk of developing. If you've been treated for one of these cancer types, you should discuss these potential, later health effects with your healthcare provider. Prompt diagnosis and treatment is very important.

GOOD ADVICE

Because post-treatment, late effects can occur long after treatment ends, this is another reason for keeping detailed records of your care. Keep a record of your radiation treatment (including how many "rads" or units of radiation you were exposed to) along with a detailed list of chemotherapy and other drugs. The American Society of Clinical Oncology (ASCO) has excellent templates for record keeping that can be used for this purpose. (See the appendix.)

BLADDER CANCER

When it comes to bladder cancers, there are no specific late effects, but you may suffer from persistent long-term effects. If you had radiation, your bladder may have shrunk, resulting in the need to urinate more frequently. You may also have urinary issues if you had to undergo surgery, and, if you underwent partial or complete surgical removal of the bladder, you may have to deal with sexual issues if nerves were damaged during the procedure.

BRAIN CANCER

Treatment for a brain tumor can have different late-term effects. Radiation or surgery can impact the brain's function. Such treatments can cause hearing loss or tinnitus (ringing in the ears), dental issues, and a wide range of thinking and memory problems. In such cases, rehabilitation can help. If the optic nerve was affected, radiation may have resulted in vision loss and, even if not, cataracts may develop years later. Emotional and behavioral changes can also occur.

BREAST CANCER

Radiation can cause heart and lung problems as well as sarcomas of blood vessels (**angiosarcomas**), bone (**osteosarcomas**), and connective tissues. These are mostly seen in the remaining breast area, chest wall, or in the arm that received radiation. This risk remains high even 30 years after treatment.

While taking tamoxifen for five years lowers the risk of recurrence in both the affected breast and unaffected breast, it increases the risk of uterine (endometrial) cancer. There is also a small risk of developing leukemia after treatment, especially if certain chemotherapy drugs were used. Lymphedema, which is arm swelling due to the removal of the underarm lymph node(s), may occur shortly after treatment or it can develop years later.

Finally, treatment also carries an increased risk of thyroid cancer, but whether this is due to radiation or tamoxifen is unknown.

COLON CANCER

Most colon cancer survivors report a good quality of life, although some are troubled with bowel issues, and those with a permanent colostomy may face social issues, including problems involving sexual intimacy, embarrassment, and other psychological and emotional issues. In addition, if you were treated for early stage colon cancer (either localized or a tumor that had invaded nearby organs) you should be carefully monitored as there is a 40 percent chance of the cancer recurrence. There is also risk of a second primary cancer in the colon or rectum.

LEUKEMIA

Adult leukemia survivors are at increased risk for a number of health problems that may occur later on depending on the type of leukemia and the type of treatment. In addition to cardiovascular disease and reduced fertility or infertility, there is also an increased risk of secondary cancers, obesity, bladder, lung and kidney damage, bone death, depression, or other psychological disorders and medical risks, such as hepatitis B and C due to blood transfusions. In addition, an increased risk of hearing loss has been found in people treated for acute myeloid leukemia (AML).

LUNG CANCER

Surgery for lung cancer may lead to impaired lung function, which can sometimes be helped by respiratory therapy and medication. Also, survivors are at risk of leukemia if certain chemotherapy drugs were used. Quitting tobacco use is essential to survivors who are smokers at risk of developing additional smoking-related cancers, particularly in the head, neck, and urinary tract.

MELANOMA

If you are a melanoma survivor, your major late-effect risk is developing additional melanomas. Studies show this is nine times more likely to happen to you due to either genetic risk factors and/or overexposure to ultraviolet radiation. For this reason, follow-up monitoring with skin care examinations is very important, as is avoiding or protecting yourself from the sun and avoiding indoor tanning beds.

NON-HODGKIN'S LYMPHOMA

Survivors of non-Hodgkin's lymphoma are at about 15 percent increased risk for several secondary types of cancer, including melanoma, Kaposi sarcoma, bone and soft tissue cancers, leukemia and myelodysplastic syndrome, as well as lung, kidney, colon, thyroid, bladder cancers, cancers of the head/neck area, and Hodgkin's disease. Treatment-related second cancer risk increases over time, and those treated when they were younger (20 years old or less) are at higher risk than those who were 70 or older when treated.

OVARIAN CANCER

Ovarian cancer survivors who carry the BRCA genes are at especially high risk of developing breast cancer, as well as some other cancers, and those with HNPCC have a high risk of colon, rectum, and small intestine cancers, as well as other cancers. Ovarian cancer survivors are also at increased risk of developing leukemia, especially if certain chemotherapy drugs were used (although this risk remains low).

SARCOMA

If you underwent radiation, you are at risk of developing lymphedema (limb swelling due to poor lymph drainage), as well as limb fracture, poor mobility, and a hardening of the soft tissues in that area, but rarely another sarcoma as a secondary cancer. Rehabilitation and medication can lessen these effects.

PROSTATE CANCER

Treating prostate cancer with radiation carries a modest risk of developing certain secondary cancers later in life, including tumors of the bladder, rectum, and the colon. Research finds this risk is lower in men who have undergone external radiation as opposed to those who opted for brachytherapy, in which radioactive "seeds" are implanted in the body.

Some studies have shown an increased risk of melanoma following either radiation or surgical removal of the prostate. Estrogen is no longer used to treat prostate cancer, but those who were recipients of estrogen therapy are at an increased risk for breast cancer.

TESTICULAR CANCER

Men treated for testicular cancer have a two to five percent probability of developing a non-treatment-related cancer in the other testicle and a recent survey found they were also at increased risk of developing prostate cancer. In terms of treatment-related cancers, survivors are twice as likely to develop a second cancer elsewhere. The risk of a solid tumor cancer is highest near the area where radiation was performed, and is most likely to occur five to 10 years or more afterwards. This risk does not diminish with time. Radiation also increases the risk of melanoma or sarcoma. The risk of leukemia (and myelodysplastic syndrome, or MDS) after treatment is also increased, but since these are rare, relatively few survivors develop them.

UTERINE CANCER

Radiation used to treat uterine cancer may increase the risk of developing bladder cancer later in life. A study in 2013 in the *BJU International* journal found that women who underwent pelvic radiation for uterine cancer to decrease the risk of recurrence were at twice the risk of developing bladder cancer during a 15-year follow-up period, and warned doctors to keep an eye out for this when treating women with this type of health history.

GOOD ADVICE

If you underwent radiation therapy, you should always protect any exposed skin in that area to help prevent the occurrence of skin cancer. This includes wearing sunscreen and protective clothing, and avoiding sunbathing and tanning beds.

Psychological Late Effects of Cancer

When you were faced with cancer, eradicating the disease quickly became your number one goal, and understandably so. Survival was of utmost importance, and little thought went into the possible side effects of life-saving treatments like chemotherapy, radiation, and surgery. Likewise, long-term emotional effects took a back seat to the issue of survival.

"When you have cancer, you just get thrown into the treatment. There's the diagnostic test, surgery, scans — you just do everything you do to get through it. You're just going, going, going, and then, finally the treatment is finished, and you're exhausted. All you can think of is, 'I want my normal life back,'" says Stacey Huber, an American Cancer Society patient resource navigator (PRN).

Or you may be surprised that once the initial euphoria over finishing treatment wears off, you feel depressed. "Many patients find that the doctors, nurses, and their fellow patients have become like family and now they feel kind of lonely, so this can be hard as well."

Although this may seem illogical, it really isn't. Many cancer patients go through it. Don't suffer in silence — talk to the professionals who helped you through your cancer. You'll find they'll be there for you afterwards as well.

FEAR OF RECURRENCE

The end of cancer treatment brings relief that is too often replaced by the fear of relapse. A cancer recurrence means the disease has returned after treatment was ended followed by a period in which no cancer cells are detectable. But cancer is known as a sneaky disease, and everyone knows someone — or more than one person — who was declared cancer-free, yet the disease returned.

Being concerned about a recurrence can be a positive motivator in that it can spur you to live a healthy lifestyle, quit detrimental habits (like smoking), and also trigger you to undergo regular screening and monitoring. But it can also be emotionally paralyzing. "Fear of recurrence is a big concern among cancer survivors," notes Dr. Catherine Hill-Kayser, a physician at the University of Pennsylvania.

For this reason, it's important to recognize that the psychological impact of cancer does not end after treatment ends. Take note of the strategies discussed in the previous chapter and note that the proactive steps, which include measures like seeing a counselor or joining a support group, are very valid and helpful post-treatment strategies. Also, talk to your cancer advocate, doctors, or others who helped you navigate treatment, as they will have post-treatment recommendations to share. Making the proactive lifestyle changes described in the next chapter is also very useful. In addition, both anxiety and post-traumatic stress disorder can manifest themselves after treatment ends, so here is information on these two important conditions.

ANXIETY

Unlike depression, anxiety is unlikely to lift after cancer treatment. Instead, anxiety can occur for the first time afterwards or, instead of diminishing, can grow stronger over the years. In fact, research shows that post-cancer treatment anxiety can occur even more strongly in couples than single people and last as long as 10 years after the cancer diagnosis. So do not hesitate to get help even if your treatment is completed; and if family members or caregivers are experiencing anxiety, make sure they get help as well.

POST-TRAUMATIC STRESS DISORDER

Post-traumatic stress disorder (PTSD) can also be viewed as an anxiety disorder. A person may develop PTSD after experiencing an extremely frightening or life-threatening situation. Although PTSD is most often associated with traumatic events such as war, sexual and physical attacks, and natural disasters, research also finds that this problem can occur in cancer patients as well.

The symptoms of PTSD are similar to those of anxiety disorder, but patients can also experience nightmares and flashbacks; avoidance of people, places, and things associated with the event; strong feelings of guilt, hopelessness, or shame; and self-destructive behavior (such as alcohol and drug abuse).

Although symptoms of PTSD usually develop within three months of the traumatic event, they can occur several months or years later. It is important that cancer patients and cancer survivors with PTSD be treated because this condition can interfere with their ability to pursue follow-up care, as well as causing an increased risk of developing other physical, mental, and social problems, leading to the loss of jobs and relationships. As with anxiety, you should also bear in mind that caregivers can develop PTSD as well.

Living Cancer-Free

WHEN ANNA STRAZZANTE LEARNED she had bladder cancer, she quickly formulated a plan that would not only carry her through her treatments, but beyond as well.

"About a year before my diagnosis, I had read the book *The Secret*, and it became my belief that I could become whatever I truly believed. So I started to think about the healthiest people I knew, and I realized they were all runners. So, at that moment, I decided that I would become a runner. I meditated on how it would feel to run a marathon and how exciting it would be to win. I started talking about it and planning for it in my mind," she recalls.

The fact that she had just been diagnosed with bladder cancer and would have her bladder removed and reconstructed did not deter Strazzante. She carried out what she intended to do and, indeed, within a few years, she had not only become a runner, but she completed the Chicago Marathon.

You don't necessarily need to become a marathon runner to live a healthy life after cancer; what you will need is to use all of the tools within your control: sticking to a nutrient-rich diet, regular exercise, and just as importantly, if not more, keeping a positive attitude. What Anne discovered in *The Secret* is the power to manifest a healthy existence using her everyday thoughts and meditations.

Remaining healthy both physically and mentally at the time of diagnosis, during treatment, and afterward is especially important because, now that an increasing number of cancer survivors are living longer, they are becoming more vulnerable to the deadly diseases that tend to be prevalent with aging, such as heart disease, diabetes, and stroke.

How Preventable Is Cancer?

The development of cancer is linked to many different things, including aging, heredity, and environmental factors such as tobacco smoke, pesticides, and other cancer-causing agents, as well as other factors we don't yet understand.

Although it's impossible to say what will prevent cancer in a specific case, many experts agree that it is possible to lessen the likelihood of developing cancer by 30 to 40 percent by taking certain preventive measures, like quitting smoking and adopting healthy lifestyle changes.

QUITTING SMOKING

Experts agree that the most important thing you can do to ensure your cancer-free survival is to quit if you still smoke or use tobacco products.

Throughout this book, you will find that smoking tobacco is associated with the development of not only lung cancer, but other cancers as well. In addition, research finds that cancer patients who smoke die sooner, and can also go on to develop secondary cancers. Therefore, quitting smoking is imperative.

Some people who smoke quit instantly when they are diagnosed with cancer, but many others chose to continue smoking, or find they cannot quit. Quitting smoking can be difficult, but today there are more tools than ever before to help you kick the habit. In addition, hospitals and treatment centers have quitting programs, including many that are tailored to cancer survivors. For links to free smoking cessation programs, see the appendix.

MAINTAINING A HEALTHY WEIGHT

It is estimated that obesity contributes to one-third of all new cancers, so experts cite maintaining a healthy weight as one of the key ways to prevent several types of cancer. Staying lean also helps guard against heart disease, high blood pressure, diabetes, and other maladies that come with aging.

The American Institute for Cancer Research (AICR) and the World Cancer Research Funds (WCRF), two organizations that jointly issue a highly-esteemed report on cancer prevention, put staying at a healthy weight on the top of their list of recommendations. This is protective against cancer in general, but especially so in guarding against cancer of the colon, uterus, kidney, and esophagus, as well as breast cancer in women who are postmenopausal, their report says.

Experts also point out that they're not just referring to the extremely obese, but those who are overweight, or even those on the heavier end of a normal weight, carry an increased risk as well.

With weight gain and obesity increasing throughout the United States, staying lean is not an easy goal. But it is a very worthwhile one and, especially if you are a cancer survivor, you should consider working with a registered dietitian or certified nutrition specialist to help you reach and stay at your goal weight.

ENGAGING IN PHYSICAL ACTIVITY

Physical activity comes second only to keeping at your goal weight when it comes to preventing cancer. Over the years, Americans have become increasingly sedentary, which not only leads to obesity, but is a potential contributing cause of cancer in itself.

The AICR/WCRF report found convincing evidence that physical activity can help prevent colon cancer, and the American Cancer Society cites some 50 studies in its conclusion that adults who are physically active cut their colon cancer risk by 30 to 40 percent, with those who are the most active reaping the highest benefit.

There is also suggestive evidence that women who are physically active have lower rates of breast cancer, and that this effect is higher in postmenopausal women, but there is some research that shows it might be true for younger women as well. There is also some evidence that suggests that physical activity may also help to protect against lung cancer, pancreatic cancer, and also some forms of aggressive prostate cancer.

But this isn't all. Because physical activity helps prevent weight gain, this adds to the types of cancers for which you are reducing your risk. You didn't fight your battle against cancer to be sidelined by other maladies, so this overwhelming evidence that physical activity is the key to preventing heart disease, diabetes, and a host of other deadly and debilitating diseases that come with aging should easily keep you in check. And lest we forget: exercise it the best way to keep your body younger longer.

Here are the AICR/WCRF's physical fitness goals to strive for:

- Be moderately physically active, equivalent to brisk walking for at least 30 minutes every day.

- As fitness improves, aim for 60 minutes or more of moderate exercise, or 30 minutes or more of vigorous physical activity every day.

- Limit sedentary habits such as watching television.

GOOD ADVICE

The American College of Sports Medicine (ACSM) offers a certification for trainers who want to work specifically with people who have been affected by cancer. A Certified Cancer Exercise Trainer (CET) is able to develop exercise programs to train clients who are going through cancer diagnosis or treatment. Visit the ACSM website at www.acsm.org to find an ACSM-certified professional.

EATING HEALTHY

The type of diet that is recommended to help cancer is the same type that has been found to reduce heart disease risk; healthy eating also translates into longevity and feeling great.

Here are some general recommendations on how to shift your diet to a healthier one. Remember, you don't have to make changes all at once — the important thing is to move in a healthier direction. The following are recommended ways to begin eating more healthfully:

Reduce Saturated Fat

Saturated fat, which is fat that typically hardens at room temperature, such as butter, lard, and the fat that marbles meat, has been linked to several different types of cancer, including breast cancer.

One recent study found that total and saturated fat intake was associated with different sub-types of breast cancer. In addition, a diet high in saturated fat is linked with obesity, which contributes to many of the cancers discussed above. A healthy way to eliminate saturated fats is to replace them with monounsaturated fats. These are fats that are liquid at room temperature but tend to solidify when chilled. These "healthy" fats include olive oil, sunflower and safflower oils, avocado, grape seed oil, peanut, and sesame oil. They are calorie-dense, though, so use them in moderation.

Reduce Your Intake of Processed Foods

There is increasing evidence that eating processed meat that contains nitrates and nitrites is — foods like hot dogs, bacon, and salami — linked with an increased risk of colon and stomach cancer. Studies have found that the more these foods are eaten, the higher the risk of cancer.

Limit Calorie-Dense Foods

Another category the AICR/WCRF study recommends steering clear of is foods and drinks that promote weight gain. These are primarily processed and packaged foods that often contain substantial amounts of sugar and fat, like cake, cookies, and other types of pastries. They also recommend against sugary drinks and fast food, noting that all these foods contribute to obesity.

Increase Your Intake of Fruits and Vegetables

Eating at least five daily servings of fruits and vegetables is a cornerstone of preventing cancer as well as heart disease, and possibly even stroke. A high intake of fruits and vegetables has been found to help protect against cancer in general, and also probably to help protect against several specific types of cancer, including the mouth, pharynx (part of throat), larynx (voice box), esophagus, stomach, lung, pancreas, and prostate, according to the AICR/ WCRF.

Fruits and vegetables are believed to reduce cancer risk in large part because of the micronutrients, including antioxidants and other bioactive compounds they contain. One particularly potent possible cancer reducer is a group of chemicals known as the carotenoids. These are found in varying concentrations in all vegetables, particularly those that are red or orange. Among the carotenoids (which are converted in the body to vitamin A) is beta-carotene, which is essential for human health; based on the recommended daily allowance of fruits, vegetables, and whole grains, as it provides about half of the vitamin A that Americans need daily.

Although research finds that beta-carotene is ineffective against many forms of cancer, there is evidence it may help protect against esophageal cancer as well as breast cancer, especially in women at high risk of it due to family history, excessive alcohol use, and ovarian cancer after menopause.

Lycopene is a carotenoid that has garnered interest because of its potential cancer preventing properties with respect to prostate, lung and stomach cancer. Lycopene is most closely associated with tomatoes, but it's also found in watermelon, red (bell) peppers, pink or red grapefruit, pink-fleshed guava, and persimmons.

Flavonoids are another group of compounds that protect against cancer, and new research suggests that one flavonoid, apigenin, could take away cancer's "superpower" to escape cell death on a molecular level. Parsley, celery, and chamomile tea are the most common sources of apigenin, but it is also found in many fruits and vegetables.

Cruciferous vegetables, like cabbage, Brussels sprouts, and kale, contain indoles, which are phytochemicals that induce the formation of enzymes believed to protect against cancer as well.

You should eat at least five servings of fruits and vegetables each day. Limit starchy vegetables and include produce of different colors, like red, green, yellow, white, purple, and orange, and also include tomatoes and tomato-based products. Don't overlook garlic, a terrific flavor enhancer that also may help protect against stomach cancer.

Supplements

Often, when people have had cancer or other serious illness, they may be tempted to over-supplement. Research that is done in laboratories may show that high-dose, nutrient supplements can be protective against or cause cancer, but the studies also show that such effects don't relate to the general population.

This is why the general rule is that you should not resort to supplements to supply the nutrients that are found in whole foods, such as fruits and vegetables. Studies that have looked at these nutrients in isolation have invariably found them to be disappointing, so most researchers believe that it is the combination of these chemicals found in whole foods that imbue them with their cancer protective effects.

Bulk Up on Fiber

Fiber is a term for compounds from plants that are not digested by the body. It is found in the outer layer of grains as well as in fruits, vegetables, legumes, and nuts.

Fiber helps add bulk to stool and helps move food more quickly through the digestive system, and for that reason is believed to help prevent colon cancer. Fiber also helps prevent heart disease, particularly by lowering the amount of so-called "bad" cholesterol in the blood. In addition, some studies find that beans and legumes may protect against stomach and prostate cancer.

Most experts recommend that adults try to eat 25 to 35 grams of fiber a day. Fiber also helps you feel satisfied, and in that way helps people lose weight. Most people think of oats and whole grains as containing fiber, but many fruits and vegetables are rich sources of fiber as well. This includes all types of beans, as well as many types of vegetables (asparagus, beets, broccoli, carrots, kale, corn, okra, and zucchini) and fruits (apples, figs, peaches, pears, prunes, raspberries, and strawberries). To bulk up fiber content, leave the skins on.

Limit Your Alcohol Intake

Alcohol consumption has been slowly rising in the United States and a recent Gallup survey shows that 67 percent of Americans imbibe. Beer remains the favorite among drinkers, followed by wine and hard liquor. But, although alcohol consumption brings about a very pleasurable effect, it is predominately composed of ethanol, which is a carcinogen. Convincing research shows that drinking alcohol is a cause of cancers of the mouth, pharynx, larynx, esophagus, colon (particularly in men), and breast, and contributes to cancer of the liver and colon cancer in women as well. Therefore, the AICR/WCRF recommends that, if alcoholic drinks are consumed, they should be limited to two drinks a day for men and one drink for women.

This is, coincidentally, the same limit on alcohol drinking that the American Heart Association recommends because, even though alcohol is considered heart protective, imbibing too much can raise the risk of blood pressure and other cardiac problems. One drink is a 12-ounce bottle of beer (4.5 percent alcohol), a five-ounce glass of wine (12 percent alcohol) or 1.5 ounces of 80-proof distilled spirits.

GOOD ADVICE

To help prevent cancer, you can put the recommendations cited above into effect, but one way to combine all of them is to follow the Mediterranean Diet. One of the most studied diets, the Mediterranean Diet has proven itself a top choice for preventing heart disease, and evidence shows it is cancer protective as well. This eating plan is rich in fruits, vegetable, high-fiber whole grains, and healthy oils. For more information on the Mediterranean Diet, see the appendix.

Herbivore or Omnivore?

Although people who eat vegetarian diets appear to be at lower risk for some forms of cancer, it's impossible to separate out the effect of going without meat from other healthful aspects of their lives. Therefore, most cancer experts do not prohibit meat, although they do recommend limiting it.

In their evaluation of research, the AICR/WCRF notes that meat is a valuable source of nutrients, particularly protein, iron, zinc, and vitamin B12. They say research shows people could eat up to 18 ounces of red meat a week without raising cancer risk. Selecting lean cuts is important (such as flank steak or extra lean ground beef).

Other good protein choices include poultry and fish. Fish is also considered heart-protective because it is rich in omega-3 fatty acids, which can help reduce both cancer and heart disease risk. Salmon, herring, and mackerel are particularly good choices.

Appendix A: Resources

Recommended Reading

Huber, Joy. *Cancer with Joy*. New York: Morgan James Publishing, 2012.

Huddleston, Peggy. *Prepare for Surgery: Guided Imagery Exercises for Relaxation and Accelerated Healing*. Cambridge, MA: Angel River Press, 2013.

Link, John D. *The Breast Cancer Survival Guide, 5th Edition*. New York: Holt, 2012.

McCallum, Jack. *The Prostate Monologues*. Emmaus, PA: Rodale, Inc., 2013.

Morra, Marion and Eva Potts. *Choices: The Complete Sourcebook for Cancer Information, Fourth Edition*. New York: Harper, 2003.

Mukherjee, Siddhartha. *The Emperor of All Maladies: A Biography of Cancer.* New York: Scribner, 2011.

Strempek Shea, Suzanne. *Songs from a Lead-Lined Room: Notes — High and Low — from My Journey through Breast Cancer and Radiation.* Boston: Beacon Press, 2003.

General Cancer Information

American Cancer Society
Tel: 800-227-2345
www.cancer.org

American Society of Clinical Oncology
Tel: 571-483-1300
www.cancer.net

National Cancer Institute
Tel: 800-4-CANCER (800-422-6237)
www.cancer.gov

National Comprehensive Care Network
This is an excellent online resource to make sure your treatment is up-to-date in accordance with the latest cancer guidelines. Click on the "Patient's Resources" tab, then "NCCN Guidelines for Patients" to find a comprehensive virtual booklet focusing on your type of cancer. There are also links on finding cancer centers, clinical trials and other information.
Tel: 215-690-0300
www.nccn.org

Stupid Cancer: The Voice of Young Adult Cancer
Tel: 877-735-4673
www.stupidcancer.org

Cancer Survivor Organizations

National Coalition for Cancer Survivorship
Tel: 877-NCCS-YES (877-622-7937)
www.canceradvocacy.org

Cancer Treatment Centers

National Cancer Institute's State-by-State Guide to Finding an NCI-Designated Cancer Treatment Center
Tel: 800-4-CANCER (800-455-6237)
www.cancer.gov/researchandfunding/extramural/cancercenters/find-a-cancer-center

Genetic and Hereditary Cancers

Force: Facing Our Risk of Cancer Empowered
Tel: 866-288-RISK (866-288-7475)
www.facingourrisk.org

Genetic Alliance
Tel: 202-966-5557
www.geneticalliance.org

National Society of Genetic Counselors
Tel: 312-321-6834
www.nsgc.org

Alternative, Complementary, and Integrative Medicine

"About Herbs" Mobile Device and Web App
Memorial Sloan Kettering Cancer Center
www.mskcc.org/cancer-care/integrative-medicine/about-herbs-botanicals-other-products

National Center for Complementary and Alternative Medicine (NCCAM)
Tel: 888-644-6226
www.nccam.nih.gov

Society for Integrative Oncology (SIO)
Tel: 347-676-1SIO
www.integrativeonc.org

Medical Associations

These organizations provide information and tools to help select and check qualifications of doctors and medical professionals:

American Board of Medical Specialties (ABMS)
Click on "Is Your Doctor Certified?"
Tel: 312-436-2600
www.abms.org

American College of Surgeons
Click on "Find a Qualified Surgeon"
Tel: 800-621-4111
www.facs.org

American Medical Association
Click on "Doctor Finder"
Tel: 800-621-8335
www.ama-assn.org/ama

Cancer Organizations by Type
BLADDER CANCER

American Bladder Cancer Society
Tel: 888-413-2344
www.bladdercancersupport.org

BRAIN CANCER

Voices Against Brain Cancer
Tel: 212-340-1340
www.voicesagainstbraincancer.org

BREAST CANCER

Breast Cancer Alliance
Tel: 203-861-0014
www.breastcanceralliance.org

National Breast Cancer Foundation
www.nationalbreastcancer.org

Sisters Network: A National African-American Breast Cancer
Survivorship Organization
Tel: 866.781.1808
www.sistersnetworkinc.org

Susan G. Komen
Tel: 877-GO-KOMEN (877-465-6636)
www.komen.org

BREAST CANCER IN MEN

John W. Nick Foundation, Inc.
Tel: 772-589-1440
www.malebreastcancer.org

COLON CANCER

Colon Cancer Alliance
Tel: 877-422-2030
www.ccalliance.org

Susie's Cause
Susan Cohen Colon Cancer Foundation
Tel: 410-244-1778
www.coloncancerfoundation.org

LEUKEMIA

Leukemia & Lymphoma Society
Tel: 914-949-5213
http://www.lls.org

MELANOMA

Melanoma Research Foundation
Tel: 800-673-1290
www.melanoma.org

NON-HODGKIN'S LYMPHOMA

Leukemia & Lymphoma Society
Tel: 914-949-5213
www.lls.org

Lymphoma Research Foundation
Tel: 212-349-2910
www.lymphoma.org/

LUNG CANCER

Lung Cancer Alliance
Tel: 800-298-2436
www.lungcanceralliance.org

Lung Cancer Research Foundation
Tel: 212-588-1580
www.lungcancerresearchfoundation.org

OVARIAN CANCER

Foundation for Women's Cancers
Tel: 800-444-4441, Tel: 312-578-1439
www.foundationforwomenscancer.org

Ovarian Cancer National Alliance
Tel: 202-331-1332
www.ovariancancer.org

PROSTATE CANCER

Prostate Cancer Foundation
Tel: 800-757-CURE (2873), 310-570-4700
www.pcf.org

SARCOMA

Sarcoma Alliance
Tel: 415-381-7236
www.sarcomaalliance.org

TESTICULAR CANCER

Testicular Cancer Society
Tel: 513-696-9827
www.testicularcancersociety.org

UTERINE CANCER

Foundation for Women's Cancers
Tel: 312-578-1439, Hotline: 800-444-4441
www.foundationforwomenscancer.org

Psychological Resources

CaringBridge
Tel: 651-452-7940
www.caringbridge.org

Children's Treehouse Foundation
Tel: 303-322-1202
www.childrenstreehousefdn.org

Kids Konnected
Tel: 949-582-5443
www.kidskonnected.org

Research Trials

ClinicalTrials.gov: A Service of the US National Institutes
of Health
www.clinicaltrials.gov

CureLauncher
Tel: 800-488-6632
www.curelauncher.com

CollabRx
Online search site for clinical trials specializing in
personalized medicine/targeted drugs
Tel: 415-248-5350
www.collabrx.com

Smoking Cessation Programs

American Cancer Society (see above)

American Lung Association
Tel: 800-LUNGUSA (800-586-4872)
www.lung.org

QuitNet
Offers community and forums to help people quit and stay
off smoking
www.quitnet.com

Support Groups and Mentoring

Check the major cancer organizations as well as associations for support groups based on specific cancers. Here are additional resources:

Cancer Care
Offers support groups for caregivers as well as for cancer patients
Tel: 800-813-HOPE (4673)
www.cancercare.org

Cancer Support Community
Tel: 202-659 -9709
www.cancersupportcommunity.org

Imerman Angels, One-on-One Cancer Support
Tel: 312-274-5529
www.imermanangels.org

Veterans

US Department of Veterans Affairs
Tel: Benefits, 800-827-1000; Healthcare, 877-888-VETS (8387)
www.publichealth.va.gov/index.asp

Appendix B: Alternative Cancer Treatments

THERE HAS BEEN PROGRESS made in the fight against cancer, but it is slow, and often the side effects of the major treatments, which include surgery, radiation, chemotherapy, are as feared — or even more feared — than the disease itself.

So it shouldn't be surprising that alternative and complimentary treatments are now a billion dollar industry. But although there are hundreds and hundreds of different types of treatments, there exists little means of evaluating them.

Even the definitions are confusing, as discussed in chapter 4. Once there were two choices; people either chose conventional cancer treatment, which basically as surgery, chemotherapy and/or radiation, or there was the alternative medicine route. But now there is a third choice, complementary, which is lumped under the acronym of "CAM." There is also a fourth variation, Integrative Medicine.

Integrative Cancer Treatment Programs

One of the hottest trends in healthcare today is the adding of "Integrative Medicine" programs to hospitals and cancer care treatment centers.

In one sense, this can be seen as smart marketing, and a way to capitalize on the $1 billion alternative medicine field. But on the other hand, this trend also benefits patients, who no longer have to go outside their cancer medical team to find these additional types of therapies, as discussed in chapter 4.

An example of this trend is the Integrative Cancer Program is the one offered at the University of Miami Miller School of Medicine's Sylvester Comprehensive Cancer Center.

All of the complementary therapies offered have been selected because they have been demonstrated to have some scientific validity, said Ashwin Mehta, M.D., who directs the program.

Within the integrative Medicine program, newly diagnosed cancer patients are schooled in how to follow a low-glycemic diet, which is low in sugar, as well as recommended to eat foods to strengthen the immune system, like fruits and vegetables, and to steer clear of fatty foods that could aggravate the body's inflammation response.

In addition, patients are screened for depression, sleep problems, and given an exercise prescription as well as recommendations on vitamins and supplements.

Also, patients (and their oncologist) have the added assurance the therapies provided won't not run counter to their recommendations, by recommending herbs, for instance, that could work counter to chemotherapy.

Alternative Health Systems

Some doctors and practitioners have developed their own specific remedies on curing cancer, but most fall under the umbrella of the following alternative healthcare systems and can be a handy way of investigating them further.

Ayurveda Medicine — A system of medicine that originated in ancient India, which is based on the principle that health depends on a balance between body, mind and spirit. This system also holds that people are comprised of elements, which, in determine how their bodies work. These include ata dosha (space and air); Pitta dosha (fire and water) and Kapha dosha (water and earth), and that good health depends on keeping these elements in balance.

Native American Healing — Native American (NA) traditional healing is identified as a whole medical system that encompasses a range of holistic treatments used by indigenous healers for a multitude of acute and chronic conditions or to promote health and wellbeing. Includes the belief in a spiritual being as well as ceremonial beliefs; the importance of being in harmony and nature; and a focus on the importance of family and community.

Naturopathy — An alternative healthcare system that is based on a belief of innate energy forces of the body that can be marshaled by natural means such as herbs, air, water, and physical means such as tissue manipulation and electrotherapy. Doctors who practice naturopathy are known as naturopathic physicians and can be recognized by the abbreviation N.D or N.M.D.

Homeopathy — Homeopathy is based on the idea that "like cures like," so medicines are comprised of substances that ordinarily could cause illness but are distilled into minute amounts that are believed to provide protection.

Holistic Medicine — Therapies intended to treat the person as a whole, rather than focus on the disease itself. Holistic medicine is intended to treat the mind, body and spirit. Treatments may include detoxification, such as colon cleansing; vitamins, body movement techniques such as tai chi

Traditional Chinese Medicine — A system of medical care that developed in China over thousands of years, which looks at the interaction between mind, body and environment, as a way of curing disease and maintaining health. Basic concepts include the Yin-yang theory, which is the concept of two opposing but complementary forces that shape the world and all life; Qi, the energy or vital life force flowing through the body; and the 5 elements (fire, earth, metal and wood), which correspond to particular organs and tissues in the body.

Diet-Based Alternative Cancer Treatments — These are treatments that hold that specific food or combinations of food can cure or treat cancer because of their particular properties. There are very many variations, but popular types include the following:

- Alkaline diet — A restrictive diet based on the theory that eliminating foods like meat, wheat and sugar will change the body's pH levels, putting it in an alkaline stat that will help eliminate cancer.

- Macrobiotic diet — Eating only unrefined foods and grains, supplemented by small amounts of vegetables.

- Superfoods — The idea that certain foods have the ability to cure or prevent cancer.

GOOD ADVICE

Be sure to find out what Integrative Medicine program is offered wherever you are treated. First, you may receive additional therapies that could bolster your health well-being, and second, you may save yourself a lot of money. Your insurance provider or Medicare will likely cover the costs, where otherwise it would have come out of your own pocket.

Electromagnetic and Energy Based Protocols

Electromagnetic therapy is form of alternative medicine that claims to treat disease by applying or pulsed electromagnetic fields (PEMF) to the body. Examples include Polarity Therapy, which is based on the theory that a negative or positive charge in a person's electromagnetic field affects their health; Magnetic therapy, which involves putting magnets on and around the body to cure disease; and Bioresonance therapy, in which electromagnetic waves are used to diagnose and treat illness.

What about Marijuana?

Marijuana has long been viewed as an alterative cancer treatment, but, although there is some clinical research that has found that cannabis (the scientific name for marijuana) may have cancer-fighting powers, it's use for this purpose remains illegal in the U.S.

However, a growing number of states — 23 as of this writing, including the District of Columbia — have approved it for use as a treatment to lessen cancer treatment-related side effects, and there are two FDA-approved drugs, dronabinol and nabilone, that are commercially made for the purpose of helping cancer patients deal with the side effects of cancer treatment.

Clinical studies have found that medical marijuana can help relieve vomiting and nausea from chemotherapy treatment, as well as stimulate appetite, relieve pain and promote better sleep.

The National Conference of State Legislators maintains a current list of the states that approve medical marijuana. For more information, see www. ncsl.org.

The National Conference of State Legislatures provides a current list of states that allow the use of medical marijuana. See www.ncsl.org.

Alternative Experts and Treatment Centers

The number of experts, treatments and clinics that offer alternative and complementary is beyond the scope of this chapter, but here is a listing of some of the most prominent, including those who offer consultation services and other that maintain highly informative websites on alternative treatments.

For an extensive state-by-state listing alternative cancer doctors, see www.cancure.org

DAVID BROWNSTEIN, M.D.

David Brownstein, M.D. is a board-certified family physician, one of the foremost practitioners of holistic medicine, and the medical director of the Center for Holistic Medicine in West Bloomfield, Mich. He is also the author of several books, along with a monthly newsletter. Dr. Brownstein believes that nutritional deficiencies, especially those involving iodine, are a chief cause of adenocarinomas, which arise from the body's glands, and are the most common form of cancer. They include breast, colon, lung and prostate cancer.

He also believes that iodine is one of the most important nutrients, a key part of the immune system and the body's first defense against cancer, and that many people who have cancer are iodine-deficient.

▶ **www.drbrownstein.com**

RUSSELL BLAYLOCK

Russell Blaylock is a neurosurgeon who is the author of three books, including over 30 scientific papers on varies topics, and three books dealing with his views on natural health, Natural Strategies for Cancer Patients, in which he discusses the ways to defeat cancer, enhance the effectiveness of conventional treatments and prevent complications associated with these treatments. He also writes Blaylock Wellness Report newsletter for Newsmax.com. He believes that conventional cancer treatments, such as chemotherapy and radiation, can damage the immune system, as well as DNA, leaving patients at risk for a second cancer. On the other hand, nonconventional treatments, especially those that deal with diet and nutrition, can fight off and prevent cancer. www.russelblaylockmd.com

▸ **www.blaylockreport.com**

DR. JOHANNA BUDWIG

Dr. Johanna Budwig of was a German biochemist, pharmacist and author who created Budwig diet o (also known as the Budwig protocol), an anti-cancer diet popularized in the 1950's. The diet, which is lacto-vegetarian, has as its cornerstone flaxseed oil combined with cottage cheese, but it also emphasizes meals rich in fiber, vegetables and fruits, and meats, while animal fats, sugar, butter and, in particular, margarine, are to be avoided. She based her diet on the theory that changing the type of fat in the diet could kill cancer cells. She died in 2003 at the age of 95, but her work is carried on at the Budwig Center in Spain, which also offers treatments.

▸ **www.budwigcenter.com**

BURTON GOLDBERG

Burton Goldberg is the author of the book "Alternative Medicine: The Definitive Guide to Cancer," as well as 17 other books and five films, including "Cancer Conquest." Goldberg treated his own bladder cancer with Chinese herbs and enzymes, and he now has early stage kidney cancer, which is in remission. He believes cancer can be put into remission using a non-sugar diet as well as non-toxic substances to bolster the immune system. He offers telephone consultations.

▸ **www.burtongoldberg.com**

JOE BROWN, N.M.D.

Dr. Brown was on track to become a conventional doctor when he was diagnosed with advanced melanoma. Believing that alternative therapies saved his life, he decided to become a naturopathic doctor and open his own clinic, where he offers a large variety of alternative therapies that can be used alone or in an integrative manner with conventional cancer treatments. His array of options is broad. On one hand, he has a large network of oncologists available for referral, and, on the other side of the spectrum, he is well-versed and can discuss alternative cancer therapies not available in the U.S.

▶ **www.doctorjoebrown.com**

STANISLAW BURZYNSKI, M.D., PH.D.

Dr. Stanislaw Burzynski is a both pioneer in alternative cancer treatment as well as being highly controversial. Since he founded his Houston clinic in 1977, Dr. Burzynski claims to have successfully treated some different 50 types of cancers, including many that are deadly, such as malignant brain tumors. The cornerstone of his treatment is a substance called "antieoplastins," which are biologically active peptides that, when inserted into the patient's genes, can cure cancer. He also uses personalized genetic testing, and, in some cases, low-dose chemotherapy. Dr. Burzynski offers a string of testimonials but he has also been the target of numerous actions by the U.S. Food and Drug Administration, as well as criticism from the National Cancer Institute, which takes issue with his claims that they are effective and also do not cause side effects.

▶ **www.burzynskiclinic.com**

JAMES FORSYTHE, M.D.

Dr. James Forsythe is both a board-certified oncologist as well as a homeopath, which is a field of alterative medicine. While he offers conventional treatment, Dr. Forsyth offers a fuller array of alternative options than do traditional cancer centers with integrative programs. Among his treatments is the Forsythe Anti-Cancer diet, which is an anti-sugar diet, along with a number of supplements, antioxidants, herbs, and vitamins. He utilizes both genetic and chemical sensitivity tests, and also believes in the value of wellness, including stress reduction, yoga, meditation, daily prayer, message and acupuncture.

▶ **www.drforsythe.com**

NICOLAS GONZALEZ, M.D.

Since his graduation from Cornell Medical School, Dr. Nicholas Gonzalez has spent much of his career working on the treatment for inoperable pancreatic cancer, but, working with Dr. Linda L. Isaacs, he also devised a treatment plan for a variety of other cancers as well. His plan includes a customized diet, supplements, and detoxification, as well as enzyme therapy in the form of a specially created pancreas product that is the cornerstone of his program. Although Dr. Gonzalez recently passed away, Dr. Isaacs is handling inquiries.

▸ **www.dr-gonzalez.com**

JOSEPH MERCOLA, M.D.

Dr. Mercola is an osteopathic physician and best selling book author who markets a number of dietary supplements and medical devices through his website. He is a leader in alternative health with a hugely influential and popular website. He no longer operates a wellness center, but his website is an excellent place to search for information on alternative practitioners thanks to the scores of interviews he has done over the years.

▸ **www.mercola.com**

RALPH MOSS, PHD.

Robert Moss, Ph.D., is a scientific writer who is also a proponent of complementary and alternative medicine. He is the author or editor of 12 books and three documentaries on topics related to cancer research and treatment, including "The Cancer Industry", "Questioning Chemotherapy," and "Customized Cancer Treatment." He currently directs the Moss Reports, which detailed reports on the 25 most common cancer diagnoses, and he also edits a monthly newsletter, ADVANCES in Cancer Treatment. He offers telephone consultations with patients not designed to replace your physician but instead to help evaluate conventional treatments, warn of scams, and offer information on credible alternatives.

▸ **www.cancerdecisions.com**

JACOB TEITELBAUM, M.D.

Dr. Jacob Teitelbaum, known also as "Dr. T," is a board-certified internist and medical director of the National Fibromyalgia and Fatigue Centers and Chronicity. He is the author of several books including "Real Cause, Real Cure," which discusses natural cure for cancer. He believes in a "comprehensive" approach to treating cancer, which incorporates both natural medicine as well as scientific based therapies. He also offers a free app entitled "Cures A-Z" that is available for both the iPhone and Android models. Check your phone's "App" store. See chapter 4 for more on "Dr. T."

▶ **www.Vitality101.com**

ANDREW WEIL, M.D.

Dr. Weil is the world-renowned guru of the natural medicine. He has appeared on the cover of Time magazine twice, and he has written many books and sold over 10 million copies. Like many alternative medicine leaders, Weil's interests are wide-ranging, and cancer is included among them. His website contains a "Cancer" channel that contains a mix of articles on conventional, integrative and alternative treatments, and he writes an informative Q&A column in which he addresses many questions on alternative cancer treatment.

▶ **www.drweil.com**

GOOD ADVICE

Just as many people are skeptical about conventional cancer treatments, there's reason to be skeptical, and it's good to be cautious about alternative treatments as well. Two watchdog organizations to check with before making your decision are the National Council Against Health Fraud and Quackwatch. They are listed in the Resource section.

JULIAN WHITAKER

Dr. Julian Whitaker is one of the foremost alternative practitioners in the U.S. He is a long-standing proponent of alternative medicine who sells a number of vitamin, supplements and other alternative cures online. He also runs the Whitaker Wellness Institute medical clinic and wellness center, which offers a number of noninvasive therapies designed to bolster the immune system and wellbeing of cancer patients during their treatment. He also publishes a monthly health newsletter.

▶ **www.whitakerwellness.com**

JUERGEN WINKLER, M.D.

Dr. Juergen Winkler's believes toxic overload is the root cause of much disease. For cancer, his approach uses a wide variety of programs, includes detoxification, nutrition, and treatments to balance and support the immune system, and also using reducing blood flow to tumors (inhibiting angiogenesis). He is also proponent of Insulin Potentiation Therapy (IPT), a therapy that combines insulin and chemotherapy. Proponents of IPT say it uses less of the chemotherapy drug, which means fewer side effects, but in a way that makes it more effective.

▶ **www.qfmed.com**

DONALD R. YANCE JR., CN, MH, RH (AHG)

Donald R. Yance Jr. is the author of several books including "Herbal Medicine Healing & Cancer" and "Adaptogens in Medical Herbalism: Elite Herbs and Natural Compounds for Mastering Stress, Aging and Chronic Disease," which is designed for health practitioners. He has devised a proprietary and therapeutic approach to healing called the Ecletic Triphasic Medical System, which is a comprehensive program that uses the fullest degree of botanical, nutritional and biomedical principals to aid in the treatment of chronic disease, including cancer. He also runs the non-profit Mederi Foundation, which personal, integrative and nutritional strategies for people living with cancer.

▶ **www.donnieyance.com**

Glossary

The following are terms that you will find in this book or hear in reference to cancer.

ablation: The removal or destruction of bodily tissue or its functioning ability.

active surveillance: A treatment plan that involves closely monitoring a patient's condition, but not administering treatment unless test results show the condition is worsening; an approach of "watching and waiting" for symptoms to present themselves or worsen, used in the treatment of certain cancers, such as prostate cancer.

acupuncture: The technique of inserting thin needles through the skin at specific points on the body to control pain and other symptoms; a type of complementary and alternative medicine.

adenocarcinoma: A common form of cancer that begins in the body's glandular cells, which are those that line certain internal organs and produce substances in the body, such as mucus, digestive juices, or other fluids; adenocarcinoma presents in most cancers of the breast, pancreas, lung, prostate, and colon.

adenoma: A benign tumor of epithelial tissue arising on a gland, and/or in epithelial tissue with glandular characteristics; epithelial tissue covers organs, glands, and other structures within the body.

adenosarcoma: A tumor that is a mixture of an adenoma (a tumor that starts on the epithelial tissue of a gland or in the gland-like cells of epithelial tissue) and a sarcoma, which is a tumor that starts in bone, cartilage, fat, muscle, blood vessels, or other connective or supportive tissue.

adjunct therapy: Another treatment used together with the primary treatment in order to assist the primary therapy; for instance, chemotherapy or radiation may be used after surgery to prevent cancer from returning; also called adjunctive therapy.

adjuvant therapy: Additional cancer treatment that is given after the primary treatment to lower the risk that the cancer will come back.

adverse effects: The term for medical problems that occur when cancer treatment affects healthy cells; also called side effects.

antigens: Substances that cause the immune system to make a specific immune response, such as a protein only found on tumor cells.

benign growths: A tumor or abnormal growth in the body that is not cancerous, which usually means it is incapable of spreading elsewhere.

biopsy: A procedure in which a piece of tissue is removed from a person's body so that it can be examined under a microscope to see if the person has cancer and, if so, what kind and how advanced it is.

bone marrow: The soft, spongy blood tissue found in the center of bones, from which blood cells are formed.

bone marrow transplant: In this procedure, bone marrow is transplanted from one individual to another, or removed from and transplanted to the same individual to replace damaged bone marrow with healthy cells. It is also used to enable an individual to withstand high doses of chemotherapy or radiation.

cancer: The overall name given to more than 100 types of diseases which are characterized by cells that are abnormal, grow, and divide quickly and often form a tumor (mass or lump). Cancer can also spread from its origin to other parts of the body. Certain kinds of cancers can grow in places like the bone marrow, where they don't form a tumor.

cancer survival rate: This term is used in conjunction with determining a cancer prognosis. It refers to the percentage of people who survive a certain type of cancer for a specific amount of time, usually five years.

cancer survivorship plan: A written document that cancer patients should receive upon finishing treatment that provides a summary of the care given and a detailed plan of ongoing care, including follow-up schedules for visits and testing, as well as recommendations for early detection and management of treatment-related effects and other health problems; may also be called a survivorship plan.

carcinoma: Cancer that starts in the skin or tissues that line or cover the internal organs.

cell: The basic structural, functional, and biological units that make up the human body.

chemotherapy: A form of cancer treatment in which drugs are used to kill cancer cells.

chemoprevention: Natural or manmade substances used to lower cancer risk. Examples include tamoxifen, an estrogen blocker for breast cancer risk, and finasteride to lower prostate cancer risk.

chromosome: A chromosome is a strand of DNA that is encoded with genes, which are the units of heredity. In most cells, humans have 22 pairs of these chromosomes plus the two sex chromosomes (XX in females and XY in males) for a total of 46.

chronic: A disease or condition that persists over a long period of time.

clear margins: Once cancerous tissue or tumor is removed, the area surrounding the removal site is thoroughly checked for remaining cancer cells. If the area is free of cancer, or demonstrates clear margins, this is a good indication that the disease has not spread.

clinical trials: Research studies that are set up using human volunteers to compare new cancer treatments with the standard or usual treatments.

complementary and alternative medicine (CAM): CAM is a term used to describe a diverse group of treatments, techniques, and products that are not considered to be conventional or standard medicine. Complementary medicine is used in addition to conventional treatments (an approach that is also called integrative medicine). Alternative therapies are unproven treatments used instead of standard treatments.

computed tomography (CT) scan: Also referred to as a CAT scan, this is a type of X-ray test that produces detailed, cross-sectional images of the body, including the soft tissues.

debulking: This refers to removing as much of a malignant tumor as possible, so that chemotherapy and/or radiation will be more effective. Debulking, or cytoreduction surgery, is often used in the case of brain or ovarian cancer.

DNA: Deoxyribonucleic acid (DNA) is the molecule that contains each individual's genetic code, which instructs every cell in the body how to develop, live, and reproduce.

gene: A gene is a single unit of genetic information, stored on twisting strands of DNA in every cell of every living being. Strands of DNA are tightly coiled together around proteins to form chromosomes; these are the basic units of heredity.

genetic testing: The analysis of a person's DNA to check for genetic mutations, or changes, that could increase the risk of cancer.

hematologist: A doctor who treats diseases of the blood. A hematologist who treats cancers of the blood is called a hematological oncologist.

hormone: A substance, such as a steroid, that is produced by an organ or gland, which courses through the body, affecting other organs or glands. Synthetic hormones can also be produced and used to act like a hormone in the body.

hormone therapy: Treatment that removes, blocks, or adds hormones to kill or slow the growth of cancer cells; also called hormonal therapy or endocrine therapy.

in situ: A Latin term that literally means "in place," and refers to a cancer that has not spread to nearby tissue; also known as "localized," or "noninvasive" cancer.

invasive cancer: Cancer that has spread beyond the tissue in which it started and has the potential to spread elsewhere in the body.

late effects: Side effects of cancer treatment that appear months or years after treatment has ended. These may include physical and mental problems, as well as development of secondary cancer.

localized cancer: Cancer that is confined to the area in which it started and has not spread elsewhere in the body; in situ, from the Latin, "in place."

lymphatic system: The network of small vessels, ducts, and organs that carry a fluid known as "lymph" throughout the body. The lymphatic system is one of the ways by which cancer can spread; part of the circulatory system which returns fluids and proteins back to the blood, also working in conjunction with the immune response to rid the body of debris and bacteria.

lymph nodes: Tiny bean-shaped organs that help fight infection and are part of the lymphatic system.

magnetic resonance imaging (MRI): This test uses radio waves and small magnets to produce detailed images of the body's soft tissue.

malignancy: A term that is synonymous with cancer that is capable of invading other tissue and spreading from one part of the body to another. Such a cancer is said to be "malignant."

mass: A lump or tumor in the body.

medical imaging: Tests and procedures that reveal internal organs and structures of the body that are hidden by the skin and bones. Types include radiography, such as X-rays, magnetic resonance imaging (MRI), positron emission tomography (PET scan) and ultrasound.

medical oncology: This is a subspecialty of internal medicine dealing with the treatment of cancers. Doctors who are medical oncologists are often the main health provider for a cancer patient. A medical oncologist may also consult with other physicians about the patient's care or refer the patient to other specialists.

metastasis: The spread of cancer from one part of the body to another.

monoclonal antibody therapy: Specialized drugs that use laboratory produced antibodies that attach to specific defects in cancer cells to help fight them.

neoadjuvant therapy: Treatment given before the main treatment, usually surgery. It may include chemotherapy, radiation therapy, or hormone therapy given prior to surgery to shrink a tumor so it is easier to remove.

oncogene: A gene that can cause cancer by promoting its growth by sending messages to the cancerous cells to grow and to spread.

oncologist: This is the name given to a doctor who specializes in the treatment of cancer.

oncology: The study of cancer.

palliative care: Treatment of the physical, spiritual, psychological, and social needs of a person with cancer. Its purpose is to improve the quality of life.

pathologist: A doctor whose specialty is studying changes in tissue and bodily fluids to diagnose disease.

polyp: A growth of normal tissue that sticks out from the lining of an organ. Some polyps can become cancerous, such as colon polyps.

positron emission tomography: Known as a PET scan, this technology is a type of nuclear medicine imaging that uses radiation to produce three-dimensional, color images of the functional processes within the human body.

precancerous: Cells that are not cancer, but could, although not always, turn into cancer. Also called premalignant.

predisposition: A tendency to develop a disease that can be triggered under certain conditions. Although a predisposition to cancer increases a person's risk of developing cancer, it is not certain that the person will develop it.

primary cancer: This term describes the original cancer. A cancer is generally described and treated in terms of the primary cancer, even if it spreads to other parts of the body.

prognosis: The outlook on the chances of surviving a disease.

radiation oncology: The use of radiation to kill cancer cells. Radiation can be done externally from a machine or performed internally by materials being put in the body near the cancerous tumor.

radiology: The use of radiation to diagnose and treat disease.

remission: The disappearance or reduction of signs of cancer upon testing. (Also termed "no evidence of cancer.") The remission can be temporary or permanent. Partial remission refers to a greater than 50 percent reduction of tumor mass.

salvage surgery: A second surgery that is performed in the event the first operation does not completely remove all signs of cancer.

screening: A test or procedure performed on an apparently healthy person to look for evidence of disease.

secondary cancer: Either a new primary cancer that develops after treatment for the first type of cancer or a cancer that has spread from the primary site to another part of the body.

side effects: Medical problems caused by cancer treatments or other medicines.

soft tissue sarcoma: A cancer that develops in the connective or supportive tissues of the body, such as the fat cells, muscle, nerves, tendons, the lining of joints, blood vessels, or lymph vessels.

stage: The classification of the extent of the cancer. Each stage of a cancer is usually grouped into a number that ranges from I to IV.

surgery: A medical operation that involves cutting open the body to remove diseased or cancerous tissue. Surgery is the most common treatment for cancer.

surgical oncologist: A specially-trained doctor who performs cancer surgery.

targeted treatment: A form of cancer therapy that takes advantage of the biologic differences between cancer cells and healthy cells by "targeting" faulty genes or proteins that contribute to cancer growth. The treatment blocks the spread of cancer cells without damaging the normal cells, thus leading to fewer side effects.

tissue: A collection of cells that work together to perform a certain job or function in the body. Different parts of the body, such as the skin, lungs, liver, or nerves, are comprised of tissue.

tumor: An abnormal mass of tissue. A tumor can be cancerous, or it can be benign, meaning it is not cancerous.

ultrasound: A diagnostic medical imaging technique used to visualize muscles, tendons, and internal organs.

Selected Bibliography

This bibliography lists the sources from which I gleaned most of my technical information, and many of my ideas and opinions on the subject of cancer, its treatment, life beyond treatment, etc. This record of sources by no means represents all of the sources that I consulted during the research and writing of this book. This selected bibliography is also meant to act as a resource that readers may consult if they are seeking additional information.

Reports

American Cancer Society. "Cancer Facts & Figures, 2014." Atlanta, GA: American Cancer Society, 2014. http://www.cancer. org/research/cancerfactsstatistics/cancerfactsfigures2014.

American Cancer Society. "Cancer Treatment & Survivorship: Facts and Figures, 2012-2013." Atlanta, GA: American Cancer Society, 2013. http://www.cancer.org/acs/groups/

content/@epidemiologysurveilance/documents/document
/acspc-033876.pdf.

Keyserlingk J, et al. "The impact treatment has on cardiovascular
risk factors for breast cancer survivors." Breast Cancer Sym-
posium, 2013; Abstract 106.

US Department of Health and Human Services, "Cancer and
Complementary Health Practices." Washington, DC: US Department of Health and Human Services, March 2012. http://
permanent.access.gpo.gov/gpo29783/Get_The_Facts_
Cancer_and_CHP_03-09-2012.pdf.

World Cancer Research Fund / American Institute for Cancer
Research. "Food, Nutrition, Physical Activity, and the Pre-
vention of Cancer: a Global Perspective." Washington, DC:
AICR, 2007. http://www.aicr.org/assets/docs/pdf/reports
/Second_Expert_Report.pdf.

Journal and Magazine Articles

American Heart Association. "Heart-healthy lifestyle also reduces cancer risk." *Science Daily*, March 18, 2013. http://www.
sciencedaily.com/releases/2013/03/130318180402.htm.

Baia, G.S., et al. "NY-ESO-1 expression in meningioma suggests
a rationale for new immunotherapeutic approaches." *Cancer
Immunology Research*, August 2013. doi:10.1158/2326-6066.

Bao, Ting, et al. "Patient-reported Outcomes in Women with
Breast Cancer Enrolled in a Dual-center, Double-blind,
Randomized Controlled Trial Assessing the effect of Acupuncture in Reducing Aromatase Inhibitor-induced Musculoskeletal Symptoms." *Cancer*, February, 2014. 120(3):
381-389.

Biel, Laura. "Biomarkers Help Patients Make Better Decisions,"
CURE, March 6, 2014. http://www.curetoday.com/
publications/cure/2014/spring2014/Biomarkers-Help-
Patients-Make-Better-Medical-Decisions.

Burkhardt, Ute E., et al. "Autologous CLL Cell Vaccination Early
After Transplant Induces Leukemia-Specific T-Cells." *Jour-
nal of Clinical Investigation*, August 5, 2013. doi: 10.1172/
JCI69098.

Brooks, Megan. "Colorectal Cancer Screening Rates Remain 'Far Too Low.'" *Medscape*, Nov. 5, 2013. http://www.medscape.com/viewarticle/813850.

Dobek, Jessica, et al. "Musculoskeletal Changes after 1 Year of Exercise in Older Breast Cancer Survivors." *Journal of Cancer Survivorship*, December 7, 2013. doi: 10.1007/s11764-013-0313-7.

Ellsworth, Rachel E. "Impact of Lifestyle Factors on Prognosis Among Breast Cancer Survivors in the USA." *Expert Reviews Pharmacoeconomics Outcomes Research*, August 2012. doi: 10.1586/erp.12.37.

Feng, JP, et al. "Secondary Diabetes Associated with 5-fluorouracil-based Chemotherapy Regimens in Non-diabetic Patients with Colorectal Cancer: Results from a Single-centre Cohort study." *Colorectal Disease*, January 2013. 15(1): 27-33.

Finch, Amy P. M. "Impact of Oophorectomy on Cancer Incidence and Mortality in Women With a BRCA1 or BRCA2 Mutation." *Journal of Clinical Oncology*, February 24, 2014. doi: 10.1200/JCO.2013.53.2820.

Florent, Cachin, et al. "123I-BZA2 as a Melanin-Targeted Radiotracer for the Identification of Melanoma Metastases: Results and Perspectives of a Multicenter Phase III Clinical Trial." *Journal of Nuclear Medicine*, November 21, 2013. doi: 10.2967/jnumed.113.123554.

Frederick, Peter and J. Michael Straughn, Jr. "The Role of Comprehensive Surgical Staging in Patients with Endometrial Cancer." *Cancer Control*, January 2009. 16(1): 23-29.

Grady, Denise. "Ovarian Cancer Study Finds Widespread Flaws in Treatment." *New York Times*, March 11, 2013. http://www.nytimes.com/2013/03/12/health/ovarian-cancer-study-finds-widespread-flaws-in-treatment.html?_r=0.

Grisham, Julie. "Studies Show Promise for Treatment Advances in Several Types of Sarcoma." *On Cancer: News and Insights from Memorial Sloan-Kettering Cancer Center*, April 22, 2013. http://www.mskcc.org/blog/studies-show-promise-treatment-advances-several-types-sarcoma.

Haslinger, Michelle, et al. "A Contemporary Analysis of Morbidity and Outcomes in Cytoreduction/Hyperthermic Intraperitoneal Chemoperfusion." *Cancer Medicine,* April 16, 2013. 2(3): 334–42.

Hildebrand, Janet S. et al. "Recreational Physical Activity and Leisure-Time Sitting in Relation to Postmenopausal Breast Cancer Risk." *Cancer Epidemiology, Biomarkers & Prevention,* October 2013. doi: 10.1158/1055-9965.EPI-13-0407.

Hill-Kayser, Christine, et al. "Impact of Internet-Based Cancer Survivorship Care Plans on Health Care and Lifestyle Behaviors." Cancer, August 6, 2013. doi: 10.1002/cncr.28286.

Horwich, A., et al. "Neoadjuvant Carboplatin before Radiotherapy in Stage IIA and IIB Seminoma." Annals of Oncology, August 2013. 24(8): 2104–7.

Johnson, George. "Why Everyone Seems to Have Cancer." *New York Times,* January 4, 2014. http://www.nytimes.com /2014/01/05/sunday-review/why-everyone-seems-to-have-cancer.html.

Kiecolt-Glaser, Janice K., et al. "Yoga's Impact on Inflammation, Mood, and Fatigue in Breast Cancer Survivors: A Randomized Controlled Trial." *Journal of Clinical Oncology,* January 27, 2014. doi:10.1200/JCO.2013.51.8860

Landro, Laura. "The Next Front in Cancer Care." *Wall Street Journal,* December 9, 2013. http://online.wsj.com/news/articles/ SB10001424052702303330204579248400281496142.

Landro, Laura. "To Treat Cancer, Treat the Distress." *Wall Street Journal,* Aug. 27, 2012. http://online.wsj.com/news /articles/SB10000872396390444914904577615291424503430.

Latour, Kathy. "Heart of the Matter: Cardiac Toxicity." *CURE,* June 17, 2013. http://www.curetoday.com/publications/cure/ 2013/summer2013/Heart-of-the-Matter-Cardiac-Toxicity.

Lee, I Min, et al. "Physical Activity and Survival After Cancer Diagnosis in Men." *Journal of Physical Activity and Health,* January 1, 2014. doi: 10.1123/jpah.2011-0257.

Li, R., et al. "Obesity, Rather Than Diet, Drives Epigenomic Alterations in Colonic Epithelium Resembling Cancer

Progression." *Cell Metabolism*, April 1, 2014. doi: 10.1016/j.cmet.2014.03.012.

Li, Wen-Qing, et al., "Personal History of Prostate Cancer and Increased History of Melanoma in the United States," *Journal of Clinical Oncology*, December 10, 2013. doi: 10.1200/JCO.2013.51.1915.

Martin, Holly, et al., "Pak and Rac GTPases Promote Oncogenic KIT-Induced Neoplasms." *Journal of Clinical Investigation*, September 16, 2013. doi: 10.1172/JCI67509.

Matjaz Rokavec, et al. "IL-6R/STAT3/miR-34a Feedback Loop Promotes EMT-mediated Colorectal Cancer Invasion and Metastasis." *Journal of Clinical Investigation*, March 2014. doi:10.1172/JCI73531.

Mirhadi, Amin, et al. "Effect of Long-Term Hormonal Therapy (vs. Short-Term Hormonal Therapy): A Secondary Analysis of Intermediate Risk Prostate Cancer Patients Treated on RTOG 9202." *International Journal of Radiation Oncology*, October 1, 2013. doi: 10.1016/j.ijrobp.2013.06.072.

Morton, Lindsay M. et al., "Stomach Cancer Risk After Treatment for Hodgkin Lymphoma," *Journal of Clinical Oncology*, September 20, 2013. 31(27): 3369-3377.

Moyer, Virginia A. "Medications for Risk Reduction of Primary Breast Cancer in Women: U.S. Preventive Services Task Force Recommendation Statement." *Annals of Internal Medicine*, September 24, 2013. http://annals.org/article.aspx?articleid=1770699.

Moyer, Virginia A., "Screening for Lung Cancer: U.S. Preventive Services Task Force Recommendation Statement." *Annals of Internal Medicine*, March 14, 2014. http://annals.org/article.aspx?articleid=1809422.

Obi, N et al. "Determinants of Newly Diagnosed Comorbidities among Breast Cancer Survivors." *Journal of Cancer Survivorship*, February 2014. 8(3); 384-93.

Ohio State University. "Compound in Mediterranean Diet Makes Cancer Cells 'Mortal.'" *ScienceDaily*, May 20, 2013. http://www.sciencedaily.com/releases/2013/05/130520154303.htm.

Parekh, Niyati. "Metabolic Dysregulation of the Insulin-Glucose Axis and Risk of Obesity-Related Cancers in the Framingham Heart Study Offspring Population 1971: 2008." *Cancer Epidemiology, Biomarkers, and Prevention*, September 24, 2013. doi: 10.1158/1055-9965.EPI-13-0330

Patel, Amish J., et al. "BET Bromodomain Inhibition Triggers Apoptosis of NF1-Associated Malignant Peripheral Nerve Sheath Tumors through Bim Induction." *Cell Reports*, 2013. doi: 10.1016/j.celrep.2013.12.001.

Reiko, Nishihara, et al. "Long-Term Colorectal Cancer Incidence and Mortality after Lower Endoscopy," *New England Journal of Medicine*, September 19, 2013. doi: 10.1056/NEJMoa1301969.

Satin, Jillian R., et al. "Depression as a Predictor of Disease Progression and Mortality in Cancer Patients: a Meta-Analysis." *Cancer*, September 14, 2009. doi: 10.1002/cncr.24561

Sieri, S., et al. "Dietary Fat Intake and Development of Specific Breast Cancer Subtypes." *Journal of the National Cancer Institute*, April 9, 2014. doi:10.1093/jnci/dju068.

Sikora, M.J. et al. "Invasive Lobular Carcinoma Cell Lines Are Characterized by Unique Estrogen-Mediated Gene Expression Patterns and Altered Tamoxifen Response." *Cancer Research*, January 14, 2014. doi: 10.1158/0008-5472.CAN-13-2779.

Singh AA, et al. "Association Between Exercise and Primary Incidence of Prostate Cancer: Does Race Matter?" *Cancer*, February 11, 2013. doi: 10.1002/cncr.27791.

Solomon, David A., et al. "Frequent Truncating Mutations of STAG2 in Bladder Cancer." *Nature Genetics*, October 13, 2013. doi: 10.1038/ng.2800.

Soneji, S., et al. "Assessing Progress in Reducing the Burden of Cancer Mortality, 1985-2005." *Journal of Clinical Oncology*, January 13, 2014. doi: 10.1200/JCO.2013.50.8952.

Sountoulides, Petros, et al. "Secondary Malignancies Following Radiotherapy for Cancer." *Therapeutic Advances in Urology*, June 1, 2010. doi: 10.1177/1756287210374462.

Stanton, Annette, et al. "Project Connect Online: Randomized Trial of an Internet-Based Program to Chronicle the Cancer Experience and Facilitate Communication." *Journal of Clinical Oncology*, September 20, 2013. doi: 10.1200/JCO.2012 .46.9015.

Stiff, Patrick J., et al. "Autologous Transplantation as Consolidation for Aggressive Non-Hodgkin's Lymphoma." *New England Journal of Medicine*, October 31, 2013. doi: 10.1056/ NEJMoa1301077.

Sukumar, Shyam, et. al. "National trends in hospital-acquired preventable adverse events after major cancer surgery in the USA." *BMJ Open*, May 1, 2013. doi: 10.1136/bmjopen -2013-002843.

Wassertheil-Smoller, et. al. "Multivitamin and Mineral Use and Breast Cancer Mortality in Older Women with Invasive Breast Cancer in the Women's Health Initiative." *Breast Cancer Research and Treatment*, 141 (3): 495-505.

Weinstein, John N., et al. "Comprehensive Molecular Characterization of Urothelial Bladder Carcinoma." *Nature*, March 20, 2014. 507(7492): 315-22.

Wiley-Blackwell. "Yoga Provides Emotional Benefits To Women With Breast Cancer." *ScienceDaily*, March 2, 2009. http:// www.sciencedaily.com/releases/2009/02/090224230707.htm.

Wu, Guan, et al. "Radiation Therapy to Treat Uterine Cancer Linked to Increased Risk of Bladder Cancer Later in Life." *BJU International*, July 17, 2014. doi: 10.1111/bju.12543.

Index

stages of, 101–102
statistics about, 98–99
TMN (tumor, node, metastases) system, 101
treatments, 103–108, 213
    active surveillance, 103–104
    brachytherapy, 107
    estrogen, 213
    external beam radiation, 107
    intensity-modulated radiation therapy (IMRT), 107
    laparoscopic prostatectomies, 105–106
    late effects of, 213
    prostatectomies, 105–106
    proton therapy, 107
    radical open prostatectomy, 105–106
    radiation therapy, 107
    robotic-assisted laparoscopic radical prostatectomy, 106
    robotic-assisted prostatectomy, 105
types of, 100
Prostate Cancer Foundation, 230
Proton therapy (proton-beam radiation therapy), 107
Proto-oncogene, 7–8 *See also* Genetics
PTSD. *See* Post-traumatic stress disorder
Pulmonary carcinoma. *See* Lung cancer

Q

QuackWatch.com, 49
Questions to ask
    about clinical trials, 38–41
    about diagnostic tests, 18, 26–27
    when selecting a doctor, 57–58
QuitNet, 231

R

Radiation therapy (radiation oncology), 29, 33–34, 52, 249
    adjuvant, 74
    external beam, 191
    heart damage from, 207–208
    intensity-modulated radiation therapy (IMRT), 107
    internal (brachytherapy), 33, 86, 104, 107, 191, 213
    intraoperative, 33
    proton therapy (proton-beam radiation therapy), 107
    radioactive "tracers," 24
    radioimmunotherapy, 34
    side effects of, 33

    skin cancer risk from, 214
    stereotactic, 116
    systemic, 33–34
    as treatment for
        bladder cancer, 127
        brain cancer, 116
        breast cancer, 74
        lung cancer, 86
        melanoma, 148
        ovarian cancer, 167
        prostate cancer, 107
        soft tissue sarcoma, 175
        testicular cancer, 183
        uterine cancer, 191
Radioimmunotherapy, 34
Radiology, 249. *See also* Imaging tests; Radiation therapy
Radon, 80
Rash, 69
rBGH. *See* Recombinant bovine growth hormone
Recombinant bovine growth hormone (rBGH), 12
Remission, 239
Research trials. *See* Clinical trials
Resectoscope, 125
Resources and support, 202–203
    alternative, complementary, and integrative medicine, 227
    general information, 226
    genetic and hereditary cancers, 227
    medical associations, 227–228
    organizations by type, 228–230
    psychological resources, 231
    recommended reading, 225–226
    research trials, 231
    smoking cessation programs, 231
    support groups and mentoring, 232
    survivor organizations, 226
    treatment centers, 227. *See also* Cancer treatment centers
    veterans, 81, 183, 232
Retrograde pyelogram, 124
Retroperitoneal lymph node dissection (RPLND), 179, 184. *See also* Testicular cancer
Rheumatoid arthritis, 152
Rituxan (rituximab), 153, 157
RPLND. *See* Retroperitoneal lymph node dissection

S

Salvage surgery, 249
Sarcoma Alliance, 230

Appendix B Index Terms

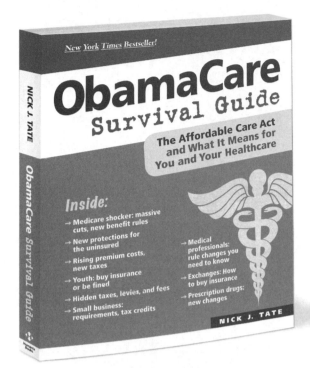

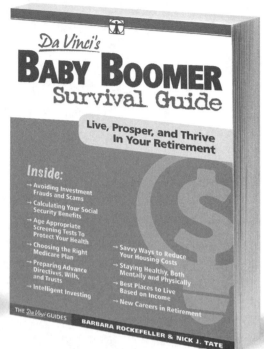

The *ObamaCare Survival Guide* reveals:

- How to maximize your healthcare dollar
- Medicare shocker: benefit cuts, new rules
- ObamaCare's impact on long-term care
- Responsibilities & penalties under new laws

Inside the *Baby Boomer Survival Guide*:

- Boost your Social Security payouts
- Health screening tests you must have
- Save money on your housing
- Best states and cities to retire in
- 10 tax tips that can save you $1,000

Own the Entire *Da Vinci* Series by Going to:

ObamaCare411.com

Boomers411.com